SELF-ASSESSMENT FOR THE MRCP: HAEMATOLOGY

SELF-ASSESSMENT FOR THE MRCP: HAEMATOLOGY

Barbara J Bain

FRACP, FRCPath

Senior Lecturer in Haematology
Imperial College School of Medicine
at St Mary's Hospital, London

Honorary Consultant Haematologist
St Mary's Hospital, London

Imperial College Press

Published by

Imperial College Press
516 Sherfield Building
Imperial College
London SW7 2AZ

Distributed by

World Scientific Publishing Co. Pte. Ltd.
P O Box 128, Farrer Road, Singapore 912805
USA office: Suite 1B, 1060 Main Street, River Edge, NJ 07661
UK office: 57 Shelton Street, Covent Garden, London WC2H 9HE

British Library Cataloguing-in-Publication Data
A catalogue record for this book is available from the British Library.

ISBN 1-86094-068-4

Printed in Singapore.

CONTENTS

Preface vii

Case Histories ("Grey Cases") 1
    Answers and Discussion 22

Data Interpretation 43
    Answers and Discussion 58

Photographs 73
    Answers and Discussion 111

PREFACE

This book has been written specifically for candidates preparing themselves for the Part 2 examination of the Royal College of Physicians. This exam has three sections: case histories (popularly referred to as "grey cases"), data interpretation and photographic questions. Fifty-five minutes are allotted for interpreting four or more case histories (one or more of which may be illustrated). Forty-five minutes are allotted for interpreting ten sets of data and 50 for interpreting 20 photographic questions (each including one or two photographs). There is a sophisticated marking system so that although only very brief answers are required the grading recognizes not only right answers and wrong answers but also adequate answers and ideal answers. In designing the questions I have tried to adhere to the format used in the MRCP examination although I have provided somewhat more information than is often given in the photographic questions. The majority of the questions have been tested on MRCP candidates at St Mary's Hospital during the last 12 to 18 months to ensure that the degree of difficulty is appropriate.

Although the format of the questions is that of the MRCP examination, this book should also be useful to candidates preparing for other similar postgraduate examinations, such as that for the Fellowship of the Royal Australasian College of Physicians. Candidates for the Part 1 examination of the Royal College of Pathologists should also find it useful. They would be expected to perform at a higher level than trainee physicians on the data interpretation and photographic questions, but might have more problems with some of the "grey cases" with a more general medical bias.

Although this book is intended to help candidates to pass examinations, I have also tried to select cases and data sets which emphasize clinically relevant information. Thus although there are some unusual conditions, of the types which appear to be popular with examiners world-wide, there are also some mundane disorders, such as iron deficiency anaemia and the anaemia of chronic disease, which are of great relevance to everyday medical practice and yet are often ill-understood. My hope is that this book will help to produce better-informed physicians rather than merely more successful examination candidates.

Barbara J. Bain, 1997

Acknowledgements

I should like to thank the examination candidates at St Mary's who tested the questions, and Dr Janice Main for reading the manuscript and making many helpful comments. I am grateful to the Audiovisual Department, Imperial College School of Medicine at St Mary's, for permission to publish Figs. 15, 33 and 36.

CASE HISTORIES ("GREY CASES")

Case History 1

A 60-year-old Caucasian bus driver complained of several episodes of dizziness, blurring of vision and paraesthesiae, each lasting 20–30 minutes. For six months he had suffered epigastric discomfort precipitated by eating and relieved by antacids. During the preceding two months he had suffered from headaches and had noted some generalized itching following hot baths. He drank no alcohol but had smoked 30–40 cigarettes per day for most of his life. He had a morning cough productive of small amounts of white sputum. He complained of some dyspnoea on exertion but was able to walk up two flights of steps to his second floor flat without stopping.

He was plethoric with conjunctival injection. There was no cyanosis or jaundice and examination of the chest was normal. There was no lymphadenopathy or other organomegaly.

The results of investigations were: WBC $15.3 \times 10^9/l$, Hb 18.5 g/dl, haematocrit 0.56, MCV 82 fl, neutrophil count $11.3 \times 10^9/l$, lymphocyte count $3.5 \times 10^9/l$, monocyte count $0.2 \times 10^9/l$, basophil count $0.3 \times 10^9/l$, platelet count $450 \times 10^9/l$, serum B_{12} 900 ng/l (normal range 165–684), red cell folate 250 µg/l (normal range 200–800), serum ferritin 15 µg/l (normal range 20–300), sodium 136 mmol/l, potassium 3.8 mmol/l, creatinine 98 µmol/l, urate 0.05 mmol/l, LDH 550 U/l (normal range 150–450), arterial oxygen saturation 95%, carboxyhaemoglobin 5%, serum erythropoietin 8 mU/ml (normal range 10–20 mU/ml).

Question

(a) What is the most likely diagnosis?

   ....

(b) What three further tests would be most useful in investigating the patient?

   ....

   ....

   ....

(c) What are the two most important aspects of management of the patient?

   ....

   ....

Case History 2

A 68-year-old woman presented with the gradual onset of fatigue and exertional dyspnoea. There was no orthopnoea or paroxysmal nocturnal dyspnoea. She had a history of ischaemic heart disease and suffered from exertional angina which had worsened recently.

   She was pale with no jaundice, lymphadenopathy, hepatosplenomegaly or bruising. The jugular venous pressure was elevated to 3 cm and there were basal crepitations and mild ankle oedema.

   The results of investigations were: WBC $9.3 \times 10^9/l$, RBC $1.82 \times 10^{12}/l$, Hb 5.5 g/dl, MCV 85 fl, platelet count $223 \times 10^9/l$, reticulocyte count 0.01%, direct antiglobulin test negative, serum iron 28 μmol/l (normal range 9–29), transferrin 3.5 g/l, serum ferritin 450 μg/l, erythrocyte sedimentation rate 40 mm/hr, serum creatinine 86 μmol/l, serum erythropoietin 125 mU/ml (normal range 5–25). The blood film showed the features of anaemia but no other abnormality.

Question

(a) What is the most likely diagnosis?

....

(b) What test would you do to confirm the diagnosis?

....

(c) Name two other tests which would be useful in elucidating the nature of the condition.

....

....

Case History 3

A 55-year-old man presented with the sudden onset of left upper quadrant and left shoulder tip pain which was worse on moving and on deep breathing. He also complained of loss of energy, fatigue, dyspnoea, anorexia, bloating, early satiety and night sweats.

He was pale and thin with mild tachycardia, mild ankle oedema and a grade I ejection systolic murmur. His hands were hot and sweaty and his temperature was 37.5°C. The spleen was tender and enlarged 15 cm below the left costal margin. There was a splenic friction rub. The liver was enlarged 2 cm below the right costal margin. There was no jaundice and no signs of liver failure.

Laboratory tests showed:

WBC	$148 \times 10^9/l$
Hb	6 g/dl
Platelet count	$550 \times 10^9/l$
Neutrophils	57%
Lymphocytes	1%
Monocytes	1%
Eosinophils	2%
Basophils	3%

Metamyelocytes	6%
Myelocytes	25%
Promyelocytes	3%
Myeloblasts	2%

Question

(a) What is the most likely diagnosis?

....

(b) What complication has occurred?

....

(c) What single test would be most useful in confirming the haematological diagnosis?

....

Case History 4

A 38-year-old known intravenous drug abuser complained of generalized weakness, a rash, arthralgia and numbness of the feet and toes. He had last used heroin 12 months previously and was maintained on methadone. Recent serological tests for HIV and hepatitis B infection had been negative.

He appeared poorly nourished and had a vasculitic rash and a distal sensory neuropathy.

Laboratory investigations showed a normal full blood count, ESR 50 mm/hr, rheumatoid factor activity present, bilirubin 15 μmol/l, aspartate transaminase 64 U/l (normal range 7–40 U/l), alanine transaminase 50 U/L (normal range < 40 IU/l), gamma GT 150 U/l (normal range < 52 IU/l). A cryoglobulin was present in a concentration of 1.6 g/l. It was composed of monoclonal IgM kappa and polyclonal IgG. C3 concentration was normal and C4 concentration reduced.

Question

(a) What is the most likely cause of the cryoglobulinaemia?

....

(b) What specific treatment might be of benefit?

....

Case History 5

A 56-year-old man presented with fatigue and diarrhoea. He was found to have iron deficiency anaemia which responded poorly to oral iron. Subsequently a jejunal biopsy was carried out and showed total villous atrophy with lamina propria infiltration by lymphocytes and plasma cells. A gluten-free diet led to symptomatic and histological improvement and a diagnosis of coeliac disease was made.

He remained on a strict gluten-free diet but two years later developed marked weight loss, abdominal pain, anorexia and diarrhoea. Laboratory investigations showed: Hb 11.2 g/dl, MCV 89 fl, ESR 40 mm/hr, serum iron 3 μmol/l (normal range 13–32 μmol/l), iron-binding capacity 19 μmol/l (45–70 μmol/l). Tests for faecal occult blood performed while the patient was on a meat-free diet were positive on three occasions. A CT scan of the abdomen showed a markedly thickened loop of jejunum.

Question

What is the most likely diagnosis?

....

Case History 6

A 70-year-old woman was referred to a rheumatologist with backache and pain in both hips. She had noted loss of height in the preceding five years. She also complained of difficulty in sleeping.

She appeared frail but not particularly unwell. There was thoracic kyphosis. The hands showed Heberden's nodes. There was no hepatomegaly, splenomegaly or lymphadenopathy.

X-rays of the chest and thoracic spine showed reduced density of thoracic vertebrae, vertebral wedging and some osteophyte formation. The heart and lung fields appeared normal. X-rays of the hips showed bilateral osteoarthritic changes. Laboratory tests showed: Hb 12 g/dl, erythrocyte sedimentation rate 60 mm in the first hour, creatinine 110 µmol/l, bilirubin 14 µmol/l, alkaline phosphatase 70 U/l (normal range 30–130 U/l), aspartate transaminase 23 U/l (normal range 7–40), total protein 83 g/l, albumin 41 g/l, calcium 2.3 mmol/l, Ig G 18 g/l (normal range 5.8–16.3), Ig A 0.9 (normal range 0.7–3.5), Ig M 0.6 g/l (normal range 0.5–2.4). The serum electrophoretic pattern showed a discrete band in the gamma region which was identified as an Ig G kappa paraprotein and was quantified at 3 g/l. A trace of Bence–Jones protein was detected in the urine. A bone marrow aspirate showed 8% plasma cells; there were occasional binucleate plasma cells.

Question

(a) What is the most likely cause of the paraproteinaemia?

....

(b) Name two further investigations which might be useful.

....

....

Case History 7

A 23-year-old woman presented with swelling and pain of the left calf. There was no other abnormality on physical examination. Doppler investigations confirmed a deep vein thrombosis extending into the popliteal and femoral veins. The patient had previously suffered two first trimester miscarriages. She was not taking the oral contraceptive or any other medication. Specific interrogation disclosed no precipitating factors for venous thrombosis. Her mother had suffered a deep vein thrombosis at the age of 75 years following a fractured hip.

The results of laboratory tests were:

WBC	$8 \times 10^9/l$
Hb	12.5 g/dl
Platelet count	$100 \times 10^9/l$
Prothrombin time	15 s (normal range 14.5–19.5)
Activated partial thromboplastin time	80 s (normal range 28–43)
Kaolin cephalin time	140 s (control 57 s)
Thrombin time	12 s (control 13 s)
Protein C activity	80% (normal range 70–148)
Free protein S antigen	85% (normal range 75–145)
Antithrombin III	105% (normal range 80–120)
Activated protein C resistance test	negative
Creatinine	67 μmol/l
Urinary protein	0.1 g/day
Urinary microscopy	normal
Antinuclear factor	negative
DNA antibodies	negative
Anticardiolipin antibodies	IgG 72 phospholipid U/ml
	IgM 13 phospholipid U/ml

Question

(a) What is the most likely diagnosis?

....

(b) What treatment should be given?

....

Case History 8

A 36-year-old man presented with a one-week history of non-specific abdominal pain. On the day of presentation the pain became severe and was associated with vomiting and diarrhoea. He complained of aching muscles and weakness. On examination he had a low grade fever and a petechial rash over the shins. There was no lymphadenopathy, hepatomegaly or splenomegaly. Heart sounds were normal. Blood pressure was 160/100. There was marked generalized abdominal tenderness. On rectal examination there was tenderness but no masses. The stools were soft, of normal colour and tested positive for blood. The urine was positive for blood and protein.

Laboratory investigations showed:

WBC	$15.3 \times 10^9/l$
Hb	16.5 g/dl
Platelet count	$400 \times 10^9/l$
Prothrombin time	16 s (normal range 14.5–19.5)
Activated partial thromboplastin time	30 s (normal range 28–43)
Thrombin time	12 s (control 13 s)
Fibrin degradation products	normal
ESR	34 mm/hr
ANA	negative
Creatinine	115 µmol/l
Bilirubin	14 µmol/l
Amylase	125 U/l (normal range 0–130)
IgG	7.8 g/l (normal range 5.8–16.3)
IgA	4.3 g/l (normal range 0.7–3.5)
IgM	1.9 g/l (normal range 0.5–2.4)
Cryoglobulins	not detected
Antistreptolysin O	negative

Computerized tomography of the abdomen showed dilated loops of small bowel and marked thickening of the wall of the jejunum.

Question

(a) What is the most likely diagnosis?

....

(b) What diagnostic procedure would you advise?

....

Case History 9

A 65-year-old man presented with a history of fatigue, weight loss, night sweats, left upper quadrant pain and early satiety. He also complained of a poor urinary stream, frequency and nocturia.

He was found to have a temperature of 37.8°C, pallor, enlargement of the liver 2 cm below the right costal margin and enlargement of the spleen 12 cm below the left costal margin. There was no lymphadenopathy. The prostate was symmetrically enlarged, smooth and firm.

Laboratory tests showed:

WBC	$3.8 \times 10^9/l$
Hb	9 g/dl
MCV	92 fl
Platelet count	$98 \times 10^9/l$
Bilirubin	18 μmol/l
Aspartate transaminase	50 U/l (normal range 7–40)
Alkaline phosphatase	450 U/l (normal range 30–130)
Calcium	2.6 mmol/l
Creatinine	98 μmol/l

The blood film showed 40% neutrophils, 58% lymphocytes, 1% monocytes, 1% myelocytes and occasional blast cells. There were two nucleated red cells to each 100 white cells. Red cells showed marked anisocytosis and poikilocytosis including some tear-drop poikilocytes and some elliptocytes.

Question

(a) What is the most likely cause of the haematological abnormalities?

....

(b) What test should be performed to confirm the diagnosis?

....

Case History 10

A four-year-old boy presented with the acute onset of fever, oliguria, pallor and jaundice. He was also suffering from bloody diarrhoea which had started six days before and was now improving. He had previously been healthy, his developmental milestones had been normal and he was fully vaccinated. His parents and seven-year-old sister were healthy. He attended a local play group and had played regularly in a local paddling pool. He had not drunk unpasteurized milk and had not eaten hamburgers in the weeks leading up to the illness.

He was found to be pale with scleral icterus and signs of fluid retention.

Laboratory investigations showed:

WBC	$14.7 \times 10^9/l$
Hb	6.5 g/dl
MCV	105 fl
Platelet count	$130 \times 10^9/l$
Neutrophil count	$13.3 \times 10^9/l$
Reticulocyte count	6.6%
Creatinine	275 μmol/l
Bilirubin	30 μmol/l
Lactic dehydrogenase	800 U/l (normal range 150–450)

The coagulation tests were normal. The blood film showed neutrophil leucocytosis with toxic granulation and vacuolation, moderate numbers of red cell fragments, polychromatic macrocytes and occasional nucleated red blood cells.

Question

(a) What is the most likely diagnosis?

....

(b) What is the most likely aetiological agent?

....

(c) Name one test which would be useful in confirming the diagnosis.

....

Case History 11

A 27-year-old woman presented with a history of the recent onset of nosebleeds and bruising.

She was found to have bruises, petechiae and an erythematous, slightly raised malar rash. Urine testing was negative for blood but showed albumin ++++.

Laboratory tests showed: WBC $3.5 \times 10^9/l$, haemoglobin 12 g/dl, MCV 87 fl, platelet count $12 \times 10^9/l$, prothrombin time 18 s (normal range 14.5–19.5), activated partial thromboplastin time 40 s (normal range 28–43), thrombin time 14 s (control 13 s), D dimer 0.1 (normal range < 0.25), antinuclear antibody positive in a titre of 160. A blood film showed few platelets, no platelet aggregates and no red cell fragments. A bone marrow aspirate showed normal granulopoiesis and erythropoiesis and plentiful megakaryocytes. Storage iron was absent.

Question

(a) What is the likely mechanism of the thrombocytopenia?

....

(b) What is the diagnosis?

....

(c) What immediate treatment would you advise?

....

Case History 12

A 73-year-old Caucasian man presented with a history where in cold weather he suffered from "poor circulation", with his lips, hands and feet going blue. On specific questioning he also reported that after episodes of cold exposure he sometimes passed pink urine. On examination the patient had generalized lymphadenopathy with nodes measuring 1–1.5 cm in diameter. The spleen was tipped on inspiration. A dipstick test for haemoglobinuria was negative.

Laboratory investigations showed: Hb 11.9 g/dl, MCV 120 fl, WBC $11.3 \times 10^9/l$, lymphocytes $5 \times 10^9/l$, platelet count $205 \times 10^9/l$, direct antiglobulin positive for complement and negative for IgG, serum haptoglobin 0.4 g/l (normal range 0.8–2.7), urinary haemosiderin positive. A blood film showed gross red cell agglutination and plasmacytoid lymphocytes.

Question

(a) What is the most likely diagnosis?

....

(b) What test would be most useful to confirm the diagnosis?

....

(c) What underlying condition is likely?

....

Case History 13

A 63-year-old woman presented with recent worsening of long term angina. She was found to have a haemoglobin concentration of 6 g/dl, MCV of 65 fl and serum ferritin of 2 µg/l (normal range 20–300). Her medical history was of appendicectomy at the age of 25 and two Caesarean sections at the ages of 27 and 29. A diagnosis of iron deficiency anaemia was made and the patient was transfused three units of packed red cells and was discharged. Ten days later she was noted to be jaundiced and was further investigated with the following results:

Bilirubin	35 µmol/l
Alanine transaminase	60 U/l (normal range < 40)
Alkaline phosphatase	64 U/l (normal range 30–130)
Serum albumin	40 g/l
Lactic dehydrogenase	500 U/l (normal range 150–450)
WBC	$11 \times 10^9/l$
Hb	7.0 g/dl
MCV	69 fl
Platelet count	$214 \times 10^9/l$

Direct antiglobulin test positive
Blood film dimorphic, hypochromic microcytes plus some spherocytes

Question

(a) What is the most likely cause of the jaundice?

....

(b) What investigation should be done?

....

(c) What are the two most important elements in the management of the patient?

....

....

Case History 14

A seven-year-old boy with short stature and mild mental retardation and with a history of pallor and bruising was referred to a paediatrician. A five-year-old sister and an 11-year-old brother were in good health, but the sister also had short stature and in addition suffered from microphthalmia. The child's mother stated that all the pregnancies had been uneventful and there was no family history of any similar congenital abnormalities in either her family or her husband's family.

On examination pallor and bruising were confirmed. There was no lymphadenopathy, hepatomegaly or splenomegaly. The child had some café-au-lait spots and some depigmented areas. Both thumbs appeared short and mispositioned.

The results of a blood count were: white cell count $3.3 \times 10^9/l$, neutrophil count $0.8 \times 10^9/l$, haemoglobin concentration 9.2 g/dl, MCV 98 fl, platelet count $85 \times 10^9/l$, reticulocyte count $10 \times 10^9/l$ (normal range 20–150). The blood film did not show any abnormality other than the pancytopenia. A bone marrow aspirate and trephine biopsy showed marked reduction of all haemopoietic lineages, with the marrow cavity being largely occupied by fat cells.

Question

(a) What is the most likely diagnosis?

....

(b) What further haematological complication may occur?

....

(c) What test should be done to confirm the diagnosis?

....

Case History 15

A 19-year-old woman presented with the recent sudden onset of moderately severe dyspnoea, dry cough and fever. She had a history of infectious mononucleosis, one year previously, and also of allergic rhinitis, but not of any other allergic disorder. She suffered from severe acne for which she had been prescribed minocycline therapy, starting two weeks before presentation. She smoked 15 cigarettes a day but did not usually have a cough or produce any sputum. She did not keep any pets and had not had any recent exposure to animals. There was no history of foreign travel.

On examination the patient appeared moderately distressed and had a fever of 39°C, basal crepitations and scattered rhonchi. Chest radiology showed bilateral basal infiltrates. A full blood count showed: WBC $14 \times 10^9/l$, haemoglobin concentration 13.3 g/dl, neutrophil count $11.6 \times 10^9/l$, eosinophil count $1.8 \times 10^9/l$, platelet count $242 \times 10^9/l$. Pulmonary function tests showed mild airways obstruction, PaO_2 7.76 kPa and CO diffusion 60% of predicted. A sputum culture grew normal flora. The serum IgE concentration was 400 µg/l (normal range 12–240).

Question

(a) What is the most likely diagnosis?

....

(b) State the three most important elements in management.

....

....

....

Case History 16

A 67-year-old Afro-Caribbean man presented with mental confusion, drowsiness and blurred vision. His wife stated that during the preceding three weeks he had complained of headaches and tiredness and had suffered a number of nosebleeds. He had been complaining of backache and pain in his ribs for about two months. There was a history of isolated atrial fibrillation which had not recurred following cardioversion two years previously. He drank 2–3 units of alcohol per day and did not smoke.

On examination the patient appeared obtunded. There was no dehydration and no stigmata of chronic liver disease. He appeared pale and had scattered bruises but no petechiae. There were no localizing neurological signs and no neck stiffness. The optic fundi showed multiple haemorrhages, soft exudates and marked venous dilation. There was no papilloedema. He was normotensive. The jugular venous pressure was elevated to 5 cm and there was mild ankle oedema. There was no hepatomegaly, splenomegaly or lymphadenopathy.

The results of initial laboratory investigations were: WBC 5.2×10^9/l, Hb 8.0 g/dl, MCV 95 fl, platelet count 120×10^9/l, bilirubin 16 µmol/l, alanine transaminase 40 IU/l (normal range < 40), alkaline phosphatase 100 U/l (normal range 30–130 U/l), total protein 100 g/l, albumin 30 g/l, calcium 2.55 mmol/l, creatinine 140 µmol/l.

Question

(a) What is the most likely cause of the patient's reduced level of consciousness and retinal abnormalities?

....

(b) What test would you request to confirm this suspicion?

....

(c) What is the most likely underlying disease?

....

(d) What single form of management is most urgently required?

....

(e) What treatment modality may be hazardous in the first instance?

....

Case History 17

A 63-year-old Indian man presented with a thrombosis of the right femoral vein. There was no family history of thrombosis, and no factors predisposing to thrombosis were identified. The patient had a six-month history of anaemia which had not responded to corticosteroids and oxymethalone and had necessitated occasional blood transfusions. There had been occasional episodes of passing dark urine but no jaundice had been noted. Serum ferritin, red cell folate and serum vitamin B_{12} concentrations had been normal when assayed prior to transfusion therapy, as were thyroid function tests and tests of liver and renal function.

On physical examination no abnormality was detected other than the signs of right femoral vein thrombosis.

Initial laboratory tests showed: WBC $4.3 \times 10^9/l$, neutrophil count $1.2 \times 10^9/l$, haemoglobin concentration 7.8 g/dl, MCV 102 fl, platelet count $50 \times 10^9/l$, reticulocyte count 7.8% ($183 \times 10^9/l$), direct antiglobulin test normal. The blood film showed only mild anisocytosis and mild polychromasia. There were no dysplastic features.

Question

(a) What is the most likely diagnosis?

....

(b) What test would you request to confirm the diagnosis?

....

(c) What is the likely nature of the anaemia?

....

(d) What two tests would you perform to confirm this?

....

....

Case History 18

A 37-year-old single man presented with the recent onset of nosebleeds. He had also noted bruising. He had previously been in good health, was teetotal, vegetarian but not vegan, did not smoke, took no medications and did not admit to any risk factors for HIV infection.

The patient appeared pale and had several large bruises which he stated had appeared spontaneously. There was no hepatomegaly, splenomegaly or lymphadenopathy. No specific lesion was identified on examination of his nose.

Initial laboratory tests showed: WBC $11.0 \times 10^9/l$, Hb 8.6 g/dl, platelet count $49 \times 10^9/l$, prothrombin time 27 s (normal range 14.5–19.5), activated partial thromboplastin time 53 s (normal range 28–32), thrombin time 22 s (control 13), fibrinogen 0.7 g/l (normal range 1.4–3.5), D-dimer > 2.0 mg/l (normal range < 0.25), FDPs > 200 mg/l (normal range < 10), blood film: normocytic, normochromic red cells; occasional blasts and promyelocytes.

An hour after the initial blood tests it was noted that the patient had bruised severely at the site of the venepuncture.

Question

(a) What is the cause of the coagulopathy?

....

(b) What is the most likely underlying diagnosis?

....

(c) What is the most important test to confirm the diagnosis?

....

Case History 19

A 73-year-old Northern European Caucasian woman who had previously been in good health presented with weight loss. On examination she was found to have enlargement of the liver to 5 cm below the costal margin; the liver was smooth, firm, regular and non-tender. There was neither jaundice nor any signs of chronic liver disease and no other abnormality was detected on physical examination. The patient drank two units of alcohol per week, did not smoke and was on no medications.

The full blood count was: WBC $9 \times 10^9/l$, Hb 13.9 g/dl, platelet count $301 \times 10^9/l$, ESR 98 mm in the first hour. A blood film showed rouleaux, Howell–Jolly bodies, acanthocytes and target cells. Biochemical investigation showed bilirubin 19 μmol/l, aspartate transaminase 103 U/l (normal range 7–40), alkaline phosphatase 585 U/l (normal range 30–130), gamma GT 491 IU/l (normal range < 52). An IgG kappa paraprotein was detected in a concentration of 21 g/l. There was no immune paresis, no free light chains were detected in the urine and a skeletal survey was normal. A bone marrow aspirate showed 10% of plasma cells which were morphologically normal. A trephine biopsy confirmed a mild diffuse increase in plasma cells. Several blood vessels showed thickening of their walls by a waxy hyaline material which stained positively with Congo red and showed apple-green birefringence on examination with polarized light.

Question

(a) What is the most likely diagnosis?

....

(b) Give two reasons for the abnormalities in the blood film.

....

....

(c) List two forms of treatment which might be of benefit.

....

....

Case History 20

A 23-year-old woman in her first pregnancy presented at 36 weeks' gestation with malaise, upper abdominal pain, nausea and vomiting. She had experienced excessive weight gain during the pregnancy and albuminuria had been recently noted. On examination she was found to have right upper quadrant tenderness, slight hepatomegaly and ankle oedema. Blood pressure was 140/90. Laboratory tests showed:

Bilirubin	30 μmol/l
Alanine transaminase	330 U/l (normal range < 40)
Alkaline phosphatase	300 U/l (normal range 30–130)
Serum albumin	28 g/l
Lactic dehydrogenase	900 U/l (normal range 150–450)
Creatinine	130 μmol/l
WBC	$21 \times 10^9/l$
Hb	9.5 g/dl
MCV	95 fl
Platelet count	$85 \times 10^9/l$
Prothrombin time	22 s (normal range 14.5–19.5)
Activated thromboplastin time	47 s (normal range 28–43)
Fibrin degradation products	20 mg/l (normal range < 10)
Fibrinogen	1.5 g/l (normal range 1.4–3.5)

The blood film showed polychromasia and moderate numbers of red cell fragments.

Question

(a) What is the most likely diagnosis?

....

(b) What are the two most important elements in management?

....

....

CASE HISTORIES ("GREY CASES")
ANSWERS AND DISCUSSION

Case 1

Answer

(a) The most likely diagnosis is polycythaemia rubra vera (primary proliferative polycythaemia).

(b) The three further tests most likely to be useful would be (i) red cell mass and plasma volume, (ii) ultrasound of the abdomen and (iii) bone marrow aspirate and trephine biopsy (possibly supplemented by cytogenetic analysis).

(c) The two most important elements in management of the patient are venesection to lower the haematocrit and advice on cessation of smoking.

Discussion

The patient has a high Hb and haematocrit. The features favouring PRV rather than any other cause of true or apparent polycythaemia are the high WBC, neutrophil count and basophil count, elevated serum B_{12} and urate concentration, low serum erythropoietin and normal oxygen saturation. The LDH is also elevated, a feature seen in about two thirds of patients with PRV. The history of itching after a hot bath favours a myeloproliferative disorder. Epigastric discomfort is present in about a third of patients with PRV and headache in about a half. Presentation with symptoms suggesting cerebrovascular disease is common. The slight reduction of the MCV and the serum ferritin concentration suggest that the patient has utilized all his body iron stores and a relative iron deficiency is limiting red cell production.

It is important to confirm that a true polycythaemia is present. A diagnosis of PRV has implications for prognosis and management of the patient, so the diagnosis must be firmly based. Ultrasound of the abdomen is useful both for the detection of splenomegaly (present in a half to three quarters of patients) and to exclude tumours or cysts of the kidneys (although the latter are unlikely as a cause of the polycythaemia in this patient given that his serum erythropoietin is low). A bone marrow aspirate and trephine biopsy are likely to show erythroid hyperplasia and sometimes also granulocytic and megakaryocytic hyperplasia. A clonal cytogenetic abnormality is present in a minority of patients, but when present is important for confirming the diagnosis. Other tests which might also be considered are (i) culture of peripheral blood mononuclear cells to detect autonomous erythroid colony growth (although the specificity of this test for myeloproliferative disorders is now doubted) and (ii) neutrophil alkaline phosphatase score (elevated in the majority of patients with PRV).

The patient should be managed by venesection to keep his haematocrit below 0.50 (and preferably below 0.45) and should be advised to stop smoking. Since his platelet count is not elevated he does not at present require cytoreductive therapy such as hydroxyurea.

Further Reading

Bilgrami, S.; Greenberg, B. R. (1995). "Polycythaemia rubra vera", *Semin. Oncol.* **22**, 307–326.

Case 2

Answer

(a) Pure red cell aplasia.

(b) Bone marrow aspirate.

(c) Chest radiography and autoantibody screen.

Discussion

The test results eliminate many causes of anaemia. There is no evidence of iron deficiency, anaemia of chronic disease or deficiency of vitamin B_{12} or folic acid. The elevation of the ESR is consistent with the age of the patient and the effect of anaemia and does not suggest an inflammatory condition. The low reticulocyte count and absence of any specific abnormality on the blood film make haemolytic anaemia unlikely and the low reticulocyte count makes haemorrhage unlikely. The myelodysplastic syndromes should be considered in a patient of this age, but the white cell count and platelet count are normal and there are no specific features to support this diagnosis. The findings are typical of pure red cell aplasia. There is a normocytic normochromic anaemia with a very low reticulocyte count and an elevated erythropoietin concentration in the serum. The absolute reticulocyte count can be calculated from the red cell count and reticulocyte percentage which are given and is $2 \times 10^9/l$ (normal range 20–150). This suggests almost complete cessation of red cell production.

The diagnosis should be confirmed by a bone marrow aspirate, which would show fairly normal cellularity but marked reduction of erythropoiesis giving a very high myeloid:erythroid ratio. Residual erythroid precursors are mainly very early forms (proerythroblasts).

The most useful tests would be radiology of the chest including a lateral view to look for a thymoma (present in 10–15% of cases of pure red cell aplasia) and an autoantibody screen. Patients with pure red cell aplasia may have autoantibodies, such as antinuclear and antithyroid antibodies. Some also have a positive direct antiglobulin test (Coombs' test). A CT scan of the chest would be an alternative to a chest X-ray, but it would seem reasonable to do a chest X-ray, as the initial radiological investigation.

If you suggested looking for antibodies to parvovirus $B_{19,}$ this is less likely to be useful since a patient without pre-existing haematological disorder (e.g. haemolytic anaemia) and with no reason to suspect impaired immunity is unlikely to have anaemia consequent on parvovirus-induced pure red cell aplasia, since such aplasia is of brief duration in subjects with normal immunity.

Case 3

Answer

(a) The most likely diagnosis is chronic granulocytic leukaemia (alternative name chronic myeloid leukaemia).

(b) The complication is splenic infarction.

(c) The single most useful test is cytogenetic analysis to detect the Philadelphia chromosome.

Discussion

The history, physical findings and differential count are all typical of chronic granulocytic leukaemia. In this type of leukaemia two cell types, myelocytes and neutrophils, predominate in the differential count. There is an absolute basophilia in virtually all cases and the majority of patients also have an absolute eosinophilia. (*Note*: if you are provided with a differential count expressed as percentages it is important to always relate this to the total white cell count in order to make a valid interpretation. The patient described has an absolute increase in both basophils and eosinophils.) An elevated platelet count as seen in this patient is common.

The symptoms and physical findings are indicative of splenic infarction.

Cytogenetic analysis is likely to reveal a specific translocation, t(9;22)(q34;q11), which gives rise to the Philadelphia chromosome. This permits a definitive diagnosis. Cytogenetic analysis is most reliable when performed on a bone marrow aspirate since there are fewer dividing cells in the blood. Bone marrow aspiration (without mention of cytogenetic analysis) or a neutrophil alkaline phosphatase (leucocyte alkaline phosphatase) score would be a less satisfactory answer to this question. A bone marrow aspirate usually shows marked granulocytic hyperplasia and increased numbers of relatively small megakaryocytes, but these changes are much less specific than the Philadelphia chromosome. Similarly, although the neutrophil alkaline phosphatase is reduced in about 95% of cases of chronic granulocytic leukaemia, it is less specific than the Philadelphia chromosome.

Further Reading

Spiers, A. S. D. (1995). "Clinical manifestations of chronic granulocytic leukaemia", *Semin. Oncol.* **22**, 380–395.

Case 4

Answer

(a) Hepatitis C infection.

(b) Interferon alpha.

Discussion

This is an example of type II mixed cryoglobulinaemia, since the cryoprecipitate contained a monoclonal and a polyclonal immunoglobulin. (In type I cryoglobulinaemia there is a monoclonal immunoglobulin which is a cryoglobulin, and in type III the cryoglobulin is polyclonal.) There is a high prevalence of hepatitis C infection in type II cryoglobulinaemia and the history of IV drug abuse in this patient makes this diagnosis very probable. Symptoms in type II cryoglobulinaemia are attributable to widespread vasculitis induced by cryoprecipitable immune complexes. Common clinical features are fatigue, arthralgia, hepatitis, glomerulonephritis and neuropathy. Early complement components such as C1q and C4 are often reduced while C3 is normal or near-normal.

Interferon alpha may be of benefit, improvement being related to a reduction in the viral load. Other, less specific therapies which may be of some use include immunosuppressive drugs, such as corticosteroids and cyclophosphamide, and plasmapheresis.

Further Reading

Agnello, V.; Chung, R. T.; Kaplan, L. M. (1992). "A role for hepatitis C virus infection in type II cryoglobulinaemia", *N. Engl. J. Med.* **327**, 1490–1495.

Misiani, R.; Bellavita, P.; Fenili, D.; Vicari, O.; Marchesi, D.; Sironi, P. L.; Zilio, P.; Vernocchi, A.; Massazza, M.; Vendramin, G.; Tanzi, E.; Zanetti, A. (1994). "Interferon alpha-2a therapy in cryoglobulinemia associated with hepatitis C virus", *N. Engl. J. Med.* **330**, 751–756.

Case 5

Answer

T-cell lymphoma of the small intestine superimposed on coeliac disease (enteropathy-associated T-cell lymphoma).

Discussion

An association of lymphoma with coeliac disease has been recognized for more than 30 years. The incidence is increased 40- to 100-fold. Lymphoma occurs mainly but not entirely in those with long-standing coeliac disease. Histologically the lesions are high grade, with large pleomorphic cells. The lesion has been misinterpreted as "malignant histiocytosis of the intestine" but more recently T-cell lineage has been confirmed. It is postulated that enteropathy-associated lymphoma emerges as a consequence of chronic T-cell activation caused by gluten hypersensitivity. A strict gluten-free diet probably offers some protection against subsequent lymphoma.

Presentation of the lymphoma may be with perforation, haemorrhage or obstruction, or there may be a recrudescence of symptoms suggestive of coeliac disease. The patient is probably suffering blood loss and in addition iron and iron-binding capacity are both reduced, a pattern seen in many patients with chronic inflammation or a malignant disease.

Further Reading

Isaacson, P. G.; O'Connor, N. T. J.; Spencer, J.; Bevan, D. H.; Connolly, C. E.; Kirkham, N.; Pollock, D. J.; Wainscoat, J. S.; Stein, H.; Mason, D. Y. (1985). "Malignant histiocytosis of the intestine: a T-cell lymphoma", *Lancet* **ii**, 688–691.

Case Records of the Massachusetts General Hospital (1996). Case 15–1996: a 79-year-old woman with anorexia, weight loss and diarrhoea after treatment for coeliac disease, *N. Engl. J. Med.* **334**, 1316–1322.

Holmes, G. K. T.; Prior, P.; Lane, M. R.; Pope, P.; Allan, R. N. (1989). "Malignancy in coeliac disease — effect of a gluten-free diet", *Gut* **30**, 333–338.

Case 6

Answer

(a) Monoclonal gammopathy of undetermined significance (MGUS). An acceptable alternative term is "benign monoclonal gammopathy".

(b) Full skeletal survey including a skull X-ray; trephine biopsy of the bone marrow.

Discussion

At least 1% of 70-year-old people have a serum paraprotein. The designation "monoclonal gammopathy of undetermined significance" is preferred to "benign monoclonal gammopathy", since not all patients continue to follow a benign clinical course. About 20% of cases develop multiple myeloma, lymphoma or other haematological malignancy within ten years. The following criteria have been suggested to make a diagnosis of MGUS rather than multiple myeloma:

> Haemoglobin concentration > 12 g/dl
> Platelet count > $150 \times 10^9/l$
> No lytic bone lesions or symptoms
> Paraprotein < 3 g/l (or Ig G paraprotein < 3.5 g/l, Ig A paraprotein < 2 g/l)
> Bence–Jones protein < 1 g/24 hr
> Bone marrow plasma cells < 10%

This patient had no anaemia, hypercalcaemia, impairment of renal function or immune paresis and appears to meet the criteria for MGUS. However, investigations are not complete. A full skeletal survey should be performed, particularly skull radiology. In addition a trephine biopsy could be useful. Multiple myeloma does not infiltrate the bone marrow in a uniform manner and a trephine biopsy sometimes reveals myeloma when the bone marrow aspirate contains less than 10% of plasma cells.

Further Reading

Kyle, R. A. (1993). "'Benign' monoclonal gammopathy: after 20–35 years of follow-up", *Mayo Clinic Proc.* **68**, 26–36.

Durie, B. G.; Clouse, I.; Braich, T.; Grimm, M.; Robertone, A. B. (1986). "Staging and kinetics of multiple myeloma", *Semin. Oncol.* **13**, 300–309.

Kyle, R. A.; Lust, J. (1989). "Monoclonal gammopathies of undetermined significance", *Semin. Hematol.* **26**, 176–200.

Baldini. L.; Guffanti, A.; Cesana, B. M.; Colombi, M.; Chiorboli, O.; Damilano, I.; Maiolo, A. T. (1996). "Role of different hematologic variables in defining the risk of malignant transformation in monoclonal gammopathy", *Blood* **87**, 912–918.

Isaksson, E.; Björkholm, M.; Holm, G.; Johansson, B.; Nilsson, B.; Mellstedt, H.; Österborg, A. (1996). "Blood clonal B-cell excess in patients with monoclonal gammopathy of undetermined significance (MGUS): association with malignant transformation", *Brit. J. Haematol.* **92**, 71–76.

Case 7

Answer

(a) Primary antiphospholipid syndrome.

(b) Heparin followed by long term warfarin.

Discussion

The occurrence of a spontaneous deep vein thrombosis in a young woman raises the possibility of inherited thrombophilia or some other underlying disorder. There was no significant family history, and tests for inherited thrombophilic disorders were negative. The prolonged activated partial thromboplastin time and kaolin cephalin time together with the history of recurrent miscarriages makes the presence of a lupus anticoagulant highly probable. This is further supported by the presence of antiphospholipid antibodies. The patient does not fit the American Rheumatism Association's criteria for systemic lupus erythematosus, the only positive feature being thrombocytopenia. The diagnosis is therefore likely to be the primary antiphospholipid syndrome. Thrombocytopenia is a common feature of this syndrome being seen in 20–40% of patients. Such patients often have negative tests for antinuclear antibodies, and antibodies to double-stranded DNA are not a feature.

Heparin is indicated for the immediate management of the patient. Since the aPTT is already prolonged it will be necessary in her case to monitor therapy by the thrombin time. She has a high titre of IgG antiphospholipid antibodies, which makes further thrombosis likely. (IgM antibodies show a weaker correlation with thrombosis.) Long term warfarin therapy is therefore indicated.

Further Reading

Asherson, R. A.; Khamashta, M. A.; Ordis-Ros, J.; Derksen, H. W. M.; Machin, S. J.; Basquinero, J.; Outt, H. H.; Harris, E. N.; Vilardell-Torres, M.; Hughes, G. R. V. (1989). "The primary antiphospholipid syndrome: major clinical and serological features", *Medicine* **68**,366–374.

Hughes, G. R. V. (1993). "The antiphospholipid syndrome: ten years on", *Lancet* **342**, 341–344.

Escalante, A.; Brey, R. L.; Mitchell, B. D.; Dreiner, U. (1995). "Accuracy of anticardiolipin antibodies in identifying a history of thrombosis among patients with systemic lupus erythematosus", *Am. J. Med.* **98**, 559–565.

Galli, M.; Finazzi, G.; Barbui, T. (1996). "Thrombocytopenia in the antiphospholipid syndrome", *Brit. J. Haematol.* **93**, 1–5.

Case 8

Answer

(a) Henoch–Schönlein purpura.

(b) Skin biopsy.

Discussion

The combination of abdominal pain, a positive test for faecal occult blood and a petechial rash on the shins is suggestive of Henoch–Schönlein purpura ("anaphylactoid purpura"). Thirty per cent of adults with Henoch–Schönlein purpura have gastrointestinal involvement.

The skin lesions are consequent on vasculitis, which may cause petechiae or palpable purpura. This diagnosis is made more likely by the elevated IgA concentration (present in 50% of patients) and the positive tests for urinary blood and protein.

A skin biopsy of a purpuric lesion is likely to be diagnostic, demonstrating vasculitis with neutrophils surrounding small vessels, IgA deposited around vessels, fibrinoid necrosis and extravasation of red cells. The IgA deposition is the most specific feature.

A renal biopsy would also be likely to confirm the diagnosis but the less invasive investigation, a skin biopsy, is preferable as the first diagnostic test.

Further Reading

Trygstad, C. W.; Stiehm, E. R. (1971). "Elevated serum IgA globulin in anaphylactoid purpura", *Pediatrics* **47**, 1023–1029.

Clinicopathologic conference (1994). "Abdominal pain, fever and rash in a 39-year-old male", *Am. J. Med.* **97**, 300–306.

Case 9

Answer

(a) Idiopathic myelofibrosis.

(b) Bone marrow trephine biopsy.

Discussion

A leucoerythroblastic blood film with hepatomegaly and marked splenomegaly suggests a diagnosis of idiopathic myelofibrosis. Acceptable alternative terminology would include "myelofibrosis with myeloid metaplasia" and "agnogenic myeloid metaplasia". In view of the marked increase of the alkaline phosphatase without much impairment of other liver function tests, it is likely that there is associated osteosclerosis.

A trephine biopsy is necessary for diagnosis. A bone marrow aspirate is likely to fail or yield only blood or a dilute non-diagnostic aspirate.

Carcinoma of the prostate is not a satisfactory answer since, although bony metastases may cause both a leucoerythroblastic blood film and elevation of the alkaline phosphatase, splenomegaly would be very unlikely. The presence of small numbers of blast cells in addition to myelocytes and nucleated red cells is also in favour of a haematological malignancy. A skeletal survey or estimation of prostate-specific antigen would be less useful, since these investigations are less likely than a trephine biopsy to lead to a specific diagnosis.

Further Reading

Tefferi, A.; Silverstein, M. N.; Noël, P. (1995). "Agnogenic myeloid metaplasia", *Sem. Oncol.* **22**, 327–333.

Case 10

Answer

(a) Haemolytic-uraemic syndrome.

(b) Verocytotoxin-producing *Escherichia coli*, particularly serotype O157.

(c) Culture of faeces on a selective medium and typing of the organism OR serological tests for antibodies to *E. coli* O157 lipopolysaccharide or to verocytotoxin.

Discussion

The blood film and count are indicative of microangiopathic haemolytic anaemia and, in view of the renal insufficiency and the history of bloody diarrhoea, the likely diagnosis is haemolytic uraemic syndrome (HUS). HUS is responsible for at least 70% of cases of acute renal failure in children in the UK. The macrocytosis is consistent with the degree of reticulocytosis. Neutrophilia and toxic changes in the neutrophils are common in HUS. Marked elevation of the neutrophil count is indicative of a worse prognosis.

In a child of this age with preceding diarrhoea the most likely cause of HUS is verocytotoxin-producing *E. coli*. Food-borne transmission is usually by beef and dairy products, including undercooked hamburgers and unpasteurized milk. Transmission may also be water-borne, by person-to-person spread and by close contact with livestock. British outbreaks have been linked to attendance at a preschool nursery and to paddling pools.

Verocytotoxin-producing *E. coli* can be selectively cultured on sorbitol MacConkey agar and then tested with an O157 antiserum. Alternatively serum can be tested for antibodies to bacterial lipopolysaccharide or to verocytotoxin.

Further Reading

Martin, D. L.; MacDonald, K. L.; White, K. E.; Soler, J. T.; Osterholm, M. T. (1990). "The epidemiology and clinical aspects of the hemolytic uremic syndrome in Minnesota", *N. Engl. J. Med.* **323**, 1161–1167.

Chart, H.; Smith, H. R.; Scotland, S. M.; Rowe, B.; Milford, D. V.; Taylor, C. M. (1991). "Serological identification of *Escherichia coli* O157:H7 infection in haemolytic uraemic syndrome", *Lancet* **337**, 138–140.

Su, C.; Brandt, L. J. (1995). "*Escherichia coli* O157:H7 infection in humans", *Ann. Intern. Med.* **123**, 698–714.

Wall, P. G.; McDonnell, R. J.; Adak, G. K.; Cheasty, T.; Smith, H. R.; Rowe, B. (1996). "General outbreaks of verocytotoxin-producing *Escherichia coli* O157 in England and Wales from 1992 to 1994", *Communicable Disease Report* **6**, R26–R33.

Case 11

Answer

(a) Immune destruction of platelets.

(b) Systemic lupus erythematosus.

(c) Corticosteroids or high dose intravenous immunoglobulin.

Discussion

The features described are indicative of autoimmune thrombocytopenic purpura as the presenting feature of systemic lupus erythematosus. The patient meets the American Rheumatism Association's criteria for a diagnosis of systemic lupus erythematosus since she has four relevant disease features: a platelet count of $<10 \times 10^9/l$, a malar rash, heavy albuminuria and a positive antinuclear antibody. Since the patient meets the criteria for a diagnosis of SLE, this is a better answer to question (b) than autoimmune thrombocytopenic purpura or idiopathic thrombocytopenic purpura. The absent bone marrow iron stores are not of any great relevance to diagnosis since this is not uncommon in young women and the patient is neither anaemic nor microcytic.

Since the patient has petechiae and a platelet count of $12 \times 10^9/l$, treatment is indicated. This would usually be oral corticosteroids, initially in a high dose, such as 40–60 mg of prednisolone daily. High dose intravenous immunoglobulin would be an acceptable alternative. Platelet transfusion would not be an acceptable answer. When there is autoimmune destruction of platelets the survival of transfused platelets will also be very short and platelet transfusion is therefore indicated only when there is serious bleeding, e.g. intracranial or major gastrointestinal bleeding.

Further Reading

Tan, E. M.; Cohen, A. S.; Fries, J. F.; Masi, A. T.; McShane D. J.; Rathfield, N. F.; Schaller, J. G.; Talal, N.; Winchester, R. J. (1982). "The 1982 revised criteria for the classification of systemic lupus erythematosus", *Arthritis Rheum.* **25**, 1271–1277.

Case 12

Answer

(a) Chronic cold haemagglutinin disease.

(b) Cold agglutinin titre and thermal amplitude.

(c) Non-Hodgkin's lymphoma.

Discussion

The findings are those of chronic cold haemagglutinin disease (CHAD). The symptoms taken in conjunction with the laboratory features indicate that the patient has a potent cold agglutinin which is causing agglutination of red cells following exposure to cold. On rewarming there is fixation of complement to the red cells, leading to red cell lysis. Such cold agglutinins are usually monoclonal IgM antibodies, and hence complement is detected on the red cells but not IgG. The low serum haptoglobin and the positive test for urinary haemosiderin indicate that the patient has suffered at least one recent episode of intravascular haemolysis, but the negative test for haemoglobinuria indicates that he was not actively haemolysing at the time of the test. The elevated MCV is likely to be factitious, since the blood film showed agglutination but there is no mention of macrocytosis. Many automated full blood counters produce a false elevation of MCV measurements in the presence of a cold agglutinin since clumps of agglutinated red cells are counted and sized as if they were single cells.

The diagnosis would be confirmed by demonstration of an increased cold agglutinin titre with the cold agglutinin showing a high thermal range.

It is very likely that this patient has an underlying lymphoproliferative disorder (non-Hodgkin's lymphoma, specifically lymphoplasmacytoid lymphoma) in view of the lymphadenopathy, peripheral blood lymphocytosis and plasmacytoid lymphocytes. The lymphoma cells would be expected to show the same light-chain restriction as the cold agglutinin.

Case 13

Answer

(a) Delayed haemolytic transfusion reaction.

(b) The causative antibody should be characterized so that, should transfusion be needed in the future, appropriate blood can be selected.

(c) The patient should be prescribed oral iron and the cause of the iron deficiency anaemia should be investigated.

Discussion

(a) The haemoglobin concentration is only slightly higher than before a three-unit blood transfusion, suggesting either that the patient is bleeding or that there has been a delayed transfusion reaction. The increased bilirubin, alanine transaminase and lactic dehydrogenase concentrations together with some spherocytes and a positive direct antiglobulin test indicate that the correct interpretation is that a delayed transfusion reaction has occurred. It is clear from the history that the patient has had at least two pregnancies and it is likely that this is the cause of the sensitization to red cell antigens. The transfusion has boosted antibody concentration from an undetectable level to a level leading to destruction of most of the transfused cells.

The antibody should be identified and the patient should be issued with a card with her blood group and information as to the antibody in case she needs further transfusion in the future.

The patient should be managed with oral iron or, if it is considered that the haemoglobin must be raised urgently, with transfusion of appropriate red cells to which she does not have antibodies. The underlying cause of the iron deficiency should be established.

Case 14

Answer

(a) Fanconi's anaemia.

(b) Acute myeloid leukaemia.

(c) Investigation to demonstrate increased chromosomal fragility.

Discussion

The history, physical findings and laboratory features are typical of Fanconi's anaemia. Cytopenia, often pancytopenia, usually develops in childhood. Inheritance is autosomal recessive. About a quarter of cases develop acute myeloid leukaemia. The diagnosis is confirmed by culturing peripheral blood lymphocytes in the presence of clastogenic agents such as diepoxybutane to demonstrate abnormal chromosomal fragility. This test should be done in all members of the sibship, since even children who lack developmental disorders may have inherited the abnormal gene and thus be susceptible to aplastic anaemia and acute myeloid leukaemia.

Case 15

Answer

(a) Minocycline-induced pulmonary infiltration with eosinophilia.

(b) Stop minocycline; administer oxygen; if severe symptoms persist, give corticosteroids.

Discussion

There are multiple causes of pulmonary infiltration with eosinophilia, including parasitic infection, hypersensitivity reactions to drugs, asthma, allergic bronchopulmonary aspergillosis and the Churg–Strauss syndrome. Minocycline-induced pulmonary infiltration with eosinophilia is well documented and commonly occurs within three weeks of starting therapy. In the absence of evidence of any other cause of the illness in this patient, a hypersensitivity reaction to this drug is the most likely diagnosis.

The most important element in management is immediate withdrawal of the drug. Patients with severe symptoms usually respond rapidly to corticosteroid therapy. Oxygen therapy may also be needed.

Further Reading

Bain, B. J.; *Blood Cells: A Practical Guide*, 2nd edition (Blackwell Science, Oxford, 1995), p. 166.

Sitbon, O.; Bidel, N.; Dussopt, C.; Azarian, R.; Braud, M. L.; Lebargy, F.; Fourme, T.; de Blay, F.; Piard, F.; Camus, P. (1994). "Minocycline pneumonitis and eosinophilia: a report on eight patients", *Arch. Intern. Med.* **154**, 1633–1640.

Case 16

Answer

(a) Hyperviscosity.

(b) Plasma viscosity (or whole blood viscosity).

(c) Multiple myeloma.

(d) Plasmapheresis.

(e) Blood transfusion.

Discussion

(a) The patient has many features which are typical of a hyperviscosity syndrome, including his neurological state, retinal changes, nosebleeds, elevated venous pressure and tiredness. There is only mild impairment of renal function and although the serum calcium (when corrected for hypoalbuminaemia) is elevated other features of hypercalcaemia are lacking; the hypercalcaemia would not explain all the clinical features. The high total protein despite a reduced serum albumin suggests that there may be a paraproteinaemia.

(b) Measurement of plasma viscosity is indicated. Symptomatic hyperviscosity caused by a paraproteinaemia is usually associated with a plasma viscosity of more than 6 mPa/s (normal range 1.5–1.72 at 25°C). Occasional cases have a lesser elevation of the plasma viscosity but the whole blood viscosity is elevated. Measurements of plasma viscosity are more widely available than measurements of whole blood viscosity and in general give at least as good separation of symptomatic and asymptomatic cases. Plasma viscosity is therefore a suitable first line test.

(c) The presence of bone pain and hypercalcaemia and the absence of hepatomegaly, splenomegaly and lymphadenopathy make multiple myeloma a more likely diagnosis than Waldenström's macroglobulinaemia. Multiple myeloma is commoner in those of African ancestry than in Northern Europeans.

(d) Plasmapheresis is urgently required.

(e) Blood transfusion may be hazardous if carried out before plasma viscosity has been lowered, since correcting the anaemia will aggravate the clinical features of hyperviscosity.

Reference

MacKenzie, M. R.; Lee, T. K. (1977). "Blood viscosity in Waldenström macroglobulinemia", *Blood* **49**, 507–510.

Case 17

Answer

(a) Paroxysmal nocturnal haemoglobinuria.

(b) Ham test (acid lysis test).

(c) Haemolytic.

(d) Serum haptoglobin concentration, urinary haemosiderin.

Discussion

The combination of an otherwise unexplained thrombotic episode with neutropenia, thrombocytopenia and anaemia with a raised reticulocyte count in a patient with a history of intermittently passing dark urine is suggestive of paroxysmal nocturnal haemoglobinuria (PNH).

The diagnosis could be confirmed by an acid lysis test (Ham test) which shows that the patient's red cells are susceptible to complement-induced lysis when the serum is acidified. An alternative test is a sugar-water test.

At some stage of the disease patients with PNH may have bone marrow hypoplasia leading to impaired red cell production and anaemia with a low reticulocyte count. In this patient there is a history suggesting haemolysis and the elevated reticulocyte count and polychromasia are indicative of a haemolytic anaemia. The mild macrocytosis is consistent with the elevated reticulocyte count.

Chronic or intermittent haemolysis can be confirmed by demonstrating a low serum haptoglobin concentration and the presence of haemosiderin in the urine (see discussion of Case 12). A study of red cell survival is not necessary and in addition it is an expensive investigation and is tedious for the patient.

Case 18

Answer

(a) Disseminated intravascular coagulation.

(b) Acute hypergranular promyelocytic leukaemia.

(c) Bone marrow aspirate with cytogenetic analysis.

Discussion

The prolonged thrombin time, reduced fibrinogen concentration and elevated concentration of D-dimer and FDPs are indicative of disseminated intravascular coagulation (DIC). Elevated fibrin degradation products alone could be consequent on primary fibrinolysis but the presence of D-dimer shows that fibrin cross-linking has occurred and is thus indicative of DIC. The history of nosebleeds, spontaneous bruises and bleeding at a venepuncture site are all consistent with DIC.

This degree of anaemia is unlikely to be consequent on nosebleeds, and the presence of occasional blasts and promyelocytes is suggestive of underlying acute leukaemia, most likely acute hypergranular promyelocytic leukaemia (M3 AML) since this sub-type is strongly associated with disseminated intravascular coagulation with associated activation of fibrinolysis.

A bone marrow aspirate is needed to confirm the diagnosis. It is of great importance that cytogenetic analysis is performed on the bone marrow aspirate in order to detect the specific translocation, t(15;17)(q22;q21), which confirms the diagnosis. Accurate diagnosis has become very important in this sub-type of acute myeloid leukaemia since the discovery that the prognosis is improved if the differentiating agent, all-trans retinoic acid (ATRA), is administered in addition to chemotherapy.

Case 19

Answer

(a) Light-chain-associated amyloidosis.

(b) Increased protein concentration (rouleaux); hyposplenism (Howell–Jolly bodies, acanthocytes, target cells).

(c) Prophylactic penicillin and appropriate vaccinations (e.g. against *Streptococcus pneumoniae, Haemophilus influenzae* type b and possibly *Neisseria meningitidis* types A and C); treatment directed at the plasma cell dyscrasia.

Discussion

(a) The bone marrow trephine biopsy showed amyloid deposition in vessel walls. The presence of slightly increased bone marrow plasma cells and a serum paraprotein indicate that it is very likely that the patient has light-chain-associated or AL amyloidosis. Primary amyloidosis would be an alternative designation. The features described do not suggest that the patient has multiple myeloma. The large smooth liver is consistent with amyloidosis and in fact a liver biopsy carried out in this patient before the diagnosis was suspected showed that the liver was infiltrated by amyloid.

(b) The blood film shows the effects of the paraprotein (which is also reflected in the high ESR) together with the features of hyposplenism. Since the patient is said to have been previously healthy and no abdominal scars were described, it is likely that the hyposplenism is consequent of splenic infiltration by amyloid.

(c) The patient should be managed like any other hyposplenic patient. Current guidelines suggest prophylactic penicillin and vaccination against pneumococcus and *Haemophilus influenzae* type b. Vaccination against meningococcus is regarded as important only when there is a high risk of exposure, for example when travelling to countries where there is a high incidence of meningococcus group A infection. The patient should also be warned about travel to areas where malaria is endemic.

There is now evidence that therapy directed specifically at the underlying plasma cell dyscrasia is of benefit although treatment with cytotoxic chemotherapy has led to some cases of myelodysplastic syndrome and secondary acute myeloid leukaemia. Intermittent melphalan could be recommended.

References

Working Party of the British Committee for Standards in Haematology Clinical Haematology Task Force (1996). "Guidelines for the prevention and treatment of infection in patients with an absent or dysfunctional spleen", *Brit. Med. J.* **312**, 430–434.

Kyle, R. A.; Greipp, P. R. (1978). "Primary systemic amyloidosis: comparison of melphalan and prednisolone versus placebo", *Blood* **52**, 818–827.

Case 20

Answer

(a) HELLP syndrome (*H*aemolysis *E*levated *L*iver enzymes *L*ow *P*latelets syndrome).

(b) Early delivery and control of hypertension.

Discussion

The clinical features and the results of laboratory tests are typical of the HELLP syndrome. This syndrome is a complication of severe pre-eclampsia or pregnancy-associated hypertension characterized by a microangiopathic haemolytic anaemia, elevated concentration of transaminases and thrombocytopenia consequent on increased platelet consumption. Twenty to forty per cent of patients have disseminated intravascular coagulation (DIC). LDH is elevated as a consequence of haemolysis. An acceptable alternative answer would be to say that the patient has microangiopathic haemolytic anaemia and platelet consumption as a consequence of pregnancy-associated hypertension.

In interpreting liver function tests in pregnant patients it should be noted that the mean serum albumin falls by about 20% during pregnancy and the mean serum alkaline phosphatase rises by two- to four-fold by the end of gestation. The plasma fibrinogen concentration also rises appreciably during pregnancy. The bilirubin and transaminase in this patient are therefore significantly elevated, but the alkaline phosphatase is not. There is evidence of DIC since there is not only thrombocytopenia but also a coagulopathy and elevated fibrin degradation products. The fibrinogen concentration does not show the elevated concentration which would be expected in pregnancy, indicating that consumption is likely to be occurring.

The most important element in management is rapid delivery of the fetus, if necessary by Caesarean section. Control of hypertension is also very important. Corticosteroids may improve platelet counts and liver function tests as well as enhancing fetal lung maturity and may be used if a decision is made that, if hypertension can be controlled, delivery should be delayed, in order to allow time for improvement in fetal lung maturity.

Further Reading

Weinstein, L. (1982). "Syndrome of hemolysis, elevated liver enzymes, and low platelet count: a severe consequence of hypertension in pregnancy", *Am. J. Obstet. Gynecol.* **142**, 159–167.

Knoz, T. A.; Olans, L. B. (1996). "Liver disease in pregnancy", *N. Engl. J. Med.* **335**, 569–576.

DATA INTERPRETATION

Question 1

A 65-year-old woman with severe rheumatoid arthritis was being treated with non-steroidal anti-inflammatory drugs and gold injections. Laboratory results were:

Hb	9.4 g/dl	
MCV	78 fl	
ESR	90 mm in first hour	
C reactive protein	11.7 mg/dl	(normal range < 0.5)
Serum iron	3 μmol/l	(normal range 9–16)
Serum transferrin	36 μmol/l	(normal range 23–38)
Serum ferritin	23 μmol/l	(normal range 10–300)

Is the patient likely to be iron-deficient?

....

Question 2

A 73-year-old woman presented with breathlessness and pallor. Laboratory tests showed:

WBC $24 \times 10^9/l$
Hb $7.6 \, g/dl$
Platelet count $400 \times 10^9/l$
Neutrophil count $7 \times 10^9/l$
Lymphocyte count $16 \times 10^9/l$
Blood film: spherocytosis, polychromatic macrocytes, smear cells
Direct antiglobulin test positive

(a) What is the most likely diagnosis?

....

(b) What complication has occurred?

....

Question 3

A 23-year-old male university student presented with fever, malaise, anorexia, acute pharyngitis, cervical lymphadenopathy and mild jaundice. Laboratory tests showed:

WBC $17.3 \times 10^9/l$
Hb $13.6 \, g/dl$
Platelet count $100 \times 10^9/l$
Neutrophil count $6.9 \times 10^9/l$
Lymphocyte count $9.8 \times 10^9/l$
Blood film: numerous atypical mononuclear cells
Paul–Bunnell screening test: negative

Name the two most likely aetiological agents.

....

....

Question 4

A 23-year-old Italian woman who had recently married had the following laboratory results:

RBC	$6.6 \times 10^{12}/l$
Hb	13.0 g/dl
Haematocrit	0.40
MCV	60 fl
MCH	19.7 pg
MCHC	32.8 g/dl
Haemoglobin A2	5.5% (normal range 2.3–3.5)
Haemoglobin F	3.0% (normal range 0.5–1.0)

(a) What is the diagnosis?

....

(b) What are the two most important elements of management?

....

....

Question 5

A 30-year-old man suffered severe soft tissue bleeding following a road traffic accident. There was no family history of abnormal bleeding. Laboratory tests showed:

Prothrombin time	18 sec	(normal range 14–19)
Activated thromboplastin time	44 sec	(normal range 28–43)
Factor VIII assay	30%	(normal range 50–150%)
Von Willebrand's antigen	75%	(normal range 50–150%)
Ristocetin cofactor	81%	(normal range 50–150%)
Bleeding time (template)	8 min	(normal range 3–10)

What is the most likely diagnosis?

....

Question 6

A patient with Crohn's disease had the following test results:

Hb	9.0 g/dl	
MCV	78 fl	
Serum iron	5.8 µmol/l	(normal range 9–16)
Transferrin	20 µmol/l	(normal range 23–38)
Ferritin	99 µm/l	(normal range 10–300)
C reactive protein	4.6 mg/dl	(normal range <0.5)
ESR	46 mm in first hour	

Is iron deficiency the most likely diagnosis?

....

Question 7

A 33-year-old woman with a family history of hereditary spherocytosis suffered the sudden onset of symptoms suggestive of severe anaemia. Laboratory tests showed:

WBC	$11.0 \times 10^9/l$,
RBC	$1.65 \times 10^{12}/l$
Hb	5.0 g/dl
MCV	85 fl
MCHC	35.3 g/dl (normal range 31.6–34.9)
Platelet count	$400 \times 10^9/l$,
Reticulocyte count	< 0.02 %
Absolute reticulocyte count	$1 \times 10^9/l$ (normal range 20–150)

The blood film showed spherocytes but no polychromasia.

(a) Is it likely that the patient has hereditary spherocytosis?

....

(b) What is the most likely cause of the acute onset of anaemia?

....

Question 8

A male infant with a history of abnormal bleeding in a maternal uncle suffered prolonged bleeding following circumcision. Laboratory tests showed:

Platelet count	275×10^9/l
Prothrombin time	15 sec (normal range 14–19)
Activated thromboplastin time	50 sec (normal range 28–43)
Thrombin time	12 sec (control 13)
Fibrinogen assay	2.3 g/l (normal range 1.4–3.5)
Factor VIII assay	75% (normal range 50–150%)
Bleeding time (Ivy)	3 min (normal range 0–4)

What is the most likely diagnosis?

....

Question 9

An 18-year-old healthy Chinese woman who was contemplating pregnancy had the following test results:

RBC	5.5×10^{12}/l
Hb	12.0 g/dl
Haematocrit	0.36
MCV	65 fl
MCH	21.8 pg
MCHC	33 g/dl
Serum ferritin	104 µg/l (normal range 20–300)
Haemoglobin A2	2.4% (normal range 2.3–3.5)
Haemoglobin F	0.6% (normal range 0.5–1.0)

(a) What is the most likely diagnosis?

....

(b) What is the significance of this diagnosis?

....

Question 10

A 50-year-old man who had previously had a prosthetic aortic valve replacement complained of breathlessness and ankle swelling, and when seen in the anticoagulant clinic was noted to be pale. Laboratory results were:

INR	3.5
Bilirubin	16 μmol/l
Aspartate transaminase	35 U/l (normal range 7–40)
Alkaline phosphatase	110 U/l (normal range 30–130)
LDH	400 U/l
Creatinine	120 μmol/l
WBC	9.8×10^9/l
Hb	10.2 g/dl
MCV	97 fl
Platelet count	336×10^{12}/l
Reticulocyte count	200×10^9/l (normal range 20–150)

Blood film: anisocytosis, poikilocytosis, fragments, occasional hypochromic cells

(a) What is the likely cause of the anaemia?

....

(b) What two tests would be most useful for confirming the diagnosis?

....

....

Question 11

A five-year-old girl presented with a history of severe nosebleeds from early infancy which had required repeated nasal packing and, on several occasions, blood transfusion. She was an only child and there was no relevant family history. The results of laboratory tests were:

WBC	$7.8 \times 10^9/l$
Hb	11.5 g/dl
Platelet count	$214 \times 10^9/l$
Blood film	normal
Prothrombin time	13 sec (normal range 14–19)
Activated thromboplastin time	32 sec (normal range 28–43)
Thrombin time	14 sec (control 13)
Bleeding time (Ivy)	20 min (normal range 0–4)

(a) What is the most likely diagnosis?

....

(b) What test would be most useful in establishing a diagnosis?

....

....

Question 12

A 40-year-old man with a history of mild epistaxis was investigated following post-appendicectomy bleeding with the following results:

Prothrombin time	15 sec (normal range 14.5–19.5)
Activated partial thromboplastin time	40 sec (normal range 28–32)
Thrombin time	14 sec (control 12)
Platelet count	$236 \times 10^9/l$
Ivy bleeding time	8 min (normal range 0–4)
Factor VIII assay	35% (normal range 50–150)

(a) What is the most likely diagnosis?

....

(b) Name two further tests which could be useful in confirmation of the diagnosis.

....

....

Question 13

A 75-year-old Caucasian female complained of fatigue and numbness of the toes. Laboratory results were:

WBC	$3.5 \times 10^9/l$
Hb	7.6 g/dl
MCV	108 fl
Platelet count	$98 \times 10^9/l$
Serum vitamin B_{12}	110 ng/l (normal range 165–684)
Red cell folate	180 µg/l (normal range 200–800)
Serum ferritin	350 µg/l (normal range 20–300)

(a) What is the most likely diagnosis?

....

(b) Name the test most likely to confirm the diagnosis.

....

(c) Name a second test which could confirm the diagnosis.

....

(d) State the likely cause of the elevated serum ferritin concentration.

....

Question 14

A 23-year-old nurse presented with the recent onset of bruising and nosebleeds. Three years earlier she had suffered a pulmonary embolus while taking an oral contraceptive and had been prescribed warfarin for three months. Otherwise she had been in good health. Her diet was good. Laboratory results were:

Hb	13.3 g/dl
Platelet count	$400 \times 10^9/l$
Prothrombin time	40 sec (normal range 14.5–19.5)
Activated partial thromboplastin time	46 sec (normal range 28–32)
Thrombin time	12 sec (control 13)
Fibrinogen	3.2 g/l (normal range 1.4–3.5)
Fibrin degradation products	5 mg/l (normal range < 10)
Bilirubin	12 μmol/l
Aspartate transaminase	30 U/l (normal range 7–40)
Alkaline phosphatase	73 U/l (normal range 30–130)

The prolonged prothrombin time and activated partial thromboplastin time were corrected by mixing with fresh normal plasma.

What is the most likely explanation of the coagulopathy?

....

Question 15

A 45-year-old Indian woman complained of lethargy and constipation. Laboratory tests showed:

WBC	$9.9 \times 10^9/l$
Hb	8.3 g/dl
MCV	85 fl
Platelet count	$249 \times 10^9/l$

Reticulocyte count	9.4%
Absolute reticulocyte count	$281 \times 10^9/l$ (normal range 20–150)
Bilirubin	32 μmol/l
Serum iron	20 μmol/l (normal range 10–30)
Total iron-binding capacity	63 μmol/l (normal range 45–70)

Blood film: basophilic stippling, polychromasia, occasional nucleated red blood cells

(a) What is the most likely diagnosis?

....

(b) What test would you request to confirm the diagnosis?

....

Question 16

A 61-year-old man presented with the sudden onset of severe back pain. He also complained of thirst and constipation. On specific questioning he stated that he had suffered from gradually increasing back pain for three months which had become acutely worse following minor exertion on the day of presentation. The patient was pale, obviously in pain and was slightly dehydrated. X-rays of the thoracic and lumbar spine showed generalized osteoporosis with wedge fractures of the third and fourth lumber vertebrae. X-rays of the pelvis showed several lytic lesions with no osteosclerotic reaction. A bone scan was normal. The results of laboratory investigations were:

WBC	$7.9 \times 10^9/l$
Hb	9.9 g/dl
MCV	87 fl
Platelet count	$148 \times 10^9/l$
ESR	30 mm/hr

Bilirubin	12 μmol/l
Aspartate transaminase	36 U/l (normal range 7–40)
Alkaline phosphatase	110 U/l (normal range 30–130)
Calcium	3.4 mmol/l
Creatinine	145 μmol/l
Total protein	60 g/l
Albumin	29 g/l
IgG	4.8 g/l (normal range 5.8–16.3)
IgA	0.5 g/l (normal range 0.7–3.5)
IgM	0.4 g/l (normal range 0.5–2.4)

(a) What is the most likely diagnosis?

....

(b) List the three tests most important in confirming the diagnosis.

....

....

....

(c) What are the two most urgent therapeutic measures?

....

....

Question 17

A 69-year-old male who had smoked 40 cigarettes a day for many years complained of intermittent claudication. He had reduced femoral, popliteal and dorsalis pedis pulses bilaterally. The spleen was not palpable. He was on no medications, was 5' 8" (1.73 m) tall and weighed 73 kg. Laboratory results were:

. WBC	$12.8 \times 10^9/l$
Neutrophil count	$9.8 \times 10^9/l$
Hb	18.0 g/dl
PCV	0.56
Platelet count	$420 \times 10^9/l$
Red cell mass	34 ml/kg (normal range 30 ± 5 ml/kg)
Plasma volume	37 ml/kg (normal range 45 ± 5 ml/kg)

(a) What is the most likely diagnosis?

....

(b) What is the most likely cause?

....

Question 18

A 60-year-old man was maintained on heparin following a femoro-popliteal bypass. Ten days postoperatively he suffered a thrombosis in his right brachial artery. Laboratory tests showed:

WBC	$11.6 \times 10^9/l$
Neutrophil count	$10 \times 10^9/l$
Hb	13.7 g/dl
Platelet count	$40 \times 10^9/l$
Activated partial thromboplastin time	80 sec (normal range 28–32)
Thrombin time	40 sec (control 13)
Fibrinogen	3.5 g/l (normal range 1.4–3.5)
FDPs	5 mg/l (normal range < 10)

(a) What is the most likely cause of the thrombocytopenia?

....

(b) What immediate action should be taken?

....

(c) What would be a likely alternative explanation of the thrombocytopenia?

....

Question 19

A 73-year-old man complaining of lethargy was found to have enlargement of the liver 3 cm below the right costal margin and of the spleen 6 cm below the left costal margin. There were no stigmata of chronic liver disease. He drank 2 pints of beer on a Saturday evening, did not smoke and was on no regular medications. Laboratory tests showed:

WBC	$23.7 \times 10^9/l$
Neutrophil count	$17.8 \times 10^9/l$
Lymphocyte count	$1.3 \times 10^9/l$
Monocyte count	$4.1 \times 10^9/l$
Eosinophil count	$0.4 \times 10^9/l$
Basophil count	$0.1 \times 10^9/l$
Hb	12.2 g/dl
MCV	107 fl
Platelet count	$110 \times 10^9/l$
ESR	15 mm/hr
Serum vitamin B_{12}	900 ng/l (normal range 210–1081)
Red cell folate	180 μg/l (normal range 145–530)
Bilirubin	14 μmol/l
Aspartate transaminase	33 U/l (normal range 7–40)

Alkaline phosphatase	88 U/l (normal range 30–130)
Gamma glutamyl transaminase	50 IU/l (normal range < 52)
Thyroid-stimulating hormone	4 mU/l (normal range 0.5–5.0)

The blood film showed anisocytosis, poikilocytosis, macrocytosis and some hypogranular and hypolobulated neutrophils (pseudo-Pelger–Hüet anomaly).

What is the most likely diagnosis?

....

Question 20

A 28-year-old HIV-positive male who had previously suffered one episode of *Pneumocystis carinii* infection presented with symptoms of anaemia. He was taking pentamidine by inhalation but no other drugs and was exposed to no known toxins. He was afebrile. Laboratory tests showed:

WBC	3.7×10^9/l
Neutrophil count	2.5×10^9/l .
Lymphocyte count	0.6×10^9/l
Hb	5.9 g/dl
MCV	93.4 fl
Platelet count	120×10^9/l
Reticulocyte count	0.1%

A bone marrow aspirate showed normal cellularity and normal numbers of megakaryocytes. Erythropoiesis was normoblastic but severely reduced. There were normal numbers of proerythroblasts but very few maturing erythroid cells.

(a) What is the likely aetiological agent?

....

(b) What test should be done for confirmation?

....

(c) What two therapeutic modalities are indicated?

....

....

DATA INTERPRETATION
ANSWERS AND DISCUSSION

Question 1

Answer

Yes, the patient is likely to be iron-deficient.

Discussion

The patient is likely to be iron-deficient (as well as having the anaemia of chronic disease). Although the transferrin and serum ferritin are both within the normal range, this combination of results is strongly suggestive of iron deficiency. Acute or chronic inflammation reduces the serum transferrin concentration whereas iron deficiency raises it. In a patient with severe rheumatoid arthritis the combination of a low serum iron and a transferrin concentration towards the upper limit of normal is strongly suggestive of iron deficiency. In addition, since the ferritin concentration is lowered by iron deficiency and elevated by acute and chronic inflammation, a ferritin which is low in the normal range despite active inflammation supports a diagnosis of iron deficiency.

Question 2

Answer

(a) Chronic lymphocytic leukaemia.

(b) Autoimmune haemolytic anaemia.

Discussion

The presence of an increased lymphocyte count with smear cells in an elderly patient suggests a diagnosis of chronic lymphocytic leukaemia. The anaemia is disproportionate to the degree of elevation of the white cell count and there is no equivalent decrease in the platelet count. This suggests that the anaemia is not consequent on bone marrow infiltration. The presence of spherocytes, polychromatic macrocytes and a positive direct antiglobulin test indicates that the patient has a complicating autoimmune haemolytic anaemia.

Question 3

Answer

Cytomegalovirus (CMV); Epstein–Barr virus (EBV).

Discussion

The clinical and laboratory features are those of infectious mononucleosis. In adults the commonest cause of heterophile antibody-negative infectious mononucleosis is CMV infection. However, only about 60% of cases of EBV-induced infectious mononucleosis have heterophile antibody at presentation, so this is also a likely diagnosis. In one series of patients about 70% of cases of heterophile-negative infectious mononucleosis were caused by CMV and about 16% by EBV. Other possible causes include toxoplasmosis and HIV infection. Both EBV and CMV infections may be associated with thrombocytopenia. About a third of patients with infectious mononucleosis have a reduced platelet count.

Further Reading

Horwitz, C. A.; Henle, W.; Henle, G.; Polesky, H.; Balfour, H. H.; Siem, R. A.; Borken, S.; Ward, P. C. J. (1977). "Heterophil-negative infectious mononucleosis and mononucleosis-like illness", *Am. J. Med.* **63**, 947–957.

Question 4

Answer

(a) Beta thalassaemia trait.

(b) Genetic counselling; avoidance of iron therapy.

Discussion

The red cell indices are strongly indicative of thalassaemia trait since there is a normal haemoglobin concentration, elevation of the red cell count and marked microcytosis. The results of haemoglobin electrophoresis indicate that this is beta thalassaemia trait since there is elevation of both haemoglobin A2 and haemoglobin F. The proportion of haemoglobin A2 is elevated in virtually all heterozygotes for beta thalassaemia and the proportion of haemoglobin F in about half. This is because delta and gamma chains, which are necessary for formation of haemoglobin A2 and haemoglobin F, are synthesized at a normal rate while the rate of synthesis of beta chains, necessary for formation of haemoglobin A, is reduced. In alpha thalassaemia trait there is no increase in the proportions of minor haemoglobins since an alpha chain is needed for formation of haemoglobins A, A2 and F. Beta thalassaemia trait has a high incidence in some parts of Italy.

Since the patient has recently married, the most important element in management is genetic counselling. In addition, iron therapy should be avoided unless iron deficiency is documented.

Question 5

Answer

Haemophilia A.

Discussion

The most likely diagnosis is haemophilia A. A low factor VIII would also be seen in von Willebrand's disease, but if this were the diagnosis abnormal results for von Willebrand's antigen, ristocetin cofactor and the bleeding time would be expected. The lack of a family history is not against the diagnosis of haemophilia A since many cases are consequent on a new mutation.

Question 6

Answer

Iron deficiency is not the most likely diagnosis.

Discussion

The most likely diagnosis is anaemia of chronic disease. Although there is a microcytic anaemia and the serum iron is low the transferrin is low, rather than high and the ferritin is normal. Inflammation can elevate the serum ferritin into the normal range, masking the effect of iron deficiency. However, the degree of elevation of the ESR does not suggest very active inflammation, and as the serum ferritin is clearly normal rather than borderline it is unlikely that there is a masked iron deficiency.

Further Reading

Kurer, S. B.; Seifert, B.; Michel, B.; Ruegg, R.; Fehr, J. (1995). "Prediction of iron deficiency in chronic inflammatory rheumatic disease anaemia", *Brit. J. Haematol.* **91**, 820–826.

Question 7

Answer

(a) Yes.

(b) Parvovirus B19-induced pure red cell aplasia.

Discussion

The blood film shows spherocytes, the MCHC is slightly elevated and the patient has a family history of hereditary spherocytosis. It is therefore very likely that she has hereditary spherocytosis. The MCHC is not always elevated in hereditary spherocytosis, so that a normal result would not have excluded this diagnosis.

The most likely explanation of the acute onset of anaemia is parvovirus B19-induced pure red cell aplasia. The lack of polychromasia and the very low reticulocyte count suggest that production of red cells has virtually stopped and because of the patient's markedly reduced red cell life-span she has become acutely anaemic. The normal MCV and normal WBC and platelet count are all in keeping with this diagnosis.

An alternative explanation would be the acute onset of megaloblastic anaemia consequent on folic acid deficiency. Patients with haemolytic anaemia have an increased requirement for folic acid and, because of the shortened red cell life span, the fall of haemoglobin concentration may be very rapid. A normal MCV does not totally exclude this diagnosis since if there is a sudden, almost complete arrest of haemopoiesis the MCV may be normal. However, the normal MCV, WBC and platelet count despite a severe anaemia make this diagnosis much less likely than parvovirus-induced pure red cell aplasia.

Question 8

Answer

Haemophilia B or factor IX deficiency.

Discussion

The most likely diagnosis is haemophilia B or factor IX deficiency (also known as Christmas disease). There is a defect in the intrinsic pathway of coagulation with no apparent abnormality of the extrinsic pathway or platelet number or function. Haemophilia A is the most common inherited defect of the intrinsic pathway but is excluded by a normal factor VIII assay. The most likely diagnosis is therefore factor IX deficiency, since this is the second-most-common inherited defect of the intrinsic pathway. The inheritance is sex-linked recessive, which is consistent with the family history.

Question 9

Answer

(a) Alpha thalassaemia trait.

(b) If the patient's partner is similarly affected, there is a significant chance of hydrops fetalis in a fetus.

Discussion

The red cell indices are strongly suggestive of thalassaemia trait. Neither iron deficiency nor anaemia of chronic disease is likely to cause severe microcytosis in the absence of anaemia. Iron deficiency is excluded by a normal serum ferritin. Beta thalassaemia and delta/beta thalassaemia are excluded by the normal haemoglobin A2 and haemoglobin F concentrations. Since alternative diagnoses are excluded, the likely diagnosis is alpha thalassaemia trait. In a Chinese woman this could be very significant. The severity of the microcytosis suggests that the woman lacks two of the four alpha genes. Chinese subjects may have alpha thalassaemia in which both alpha genes are missing from a single chromosome. If this is so in the patient and her partner, then the chance of hydrops fetalis is 25%.

Question 10

Answer

(a) Mechanical haemolytic anaemia consequent on a malfunctioning prosthetic valve.

(b) Serum haptoglobin concentration; urinary haemosiderin.

Discussion

The presence of anaemia, a raised reticulocyte count and red cell fragments suggests a diagnosis of mechanical haemolytic anaemia. The lack of any elevation of the bilirubin and LDH is not inconsistent with this diagnosis since haemolysis is intravascular. An alternative diagnosis which should be considered is blood loss, even though the patient's

INR is within the therapeutic range. However, although blood loss would explain anaemia and polychromasia it would not explain the presence of red cell fragments.

Serum haptoglobin would be expected to be very low or absent in this patient since intravascular haemolysis leads to formation of haemoglobin–haptoglobin complexes which are removed by the liver. Once haptoglobin is fully saturated any further release of haemoglobin from fragmentation of red cells leads to loss of haemoglobin in the urine. Excreted haemoglobin is taken up by renal tubular cells and converted to haemosiderin. Subsequently renal tubular cells are shed in the urine so that haemosiderin is detectable in the urine.

These two tests would be the most useful investigations in this patient since they demonstrate that intravascular haemolysis is occurring. Estimation of red cell survival would be less useful since a decreased red cell life span merely confirms the haemolysis without further elucidating its cause. In addition, this test is more expensive and time-consuming. Investigation of the function of the prosthetic valve is also indicated.

Question 11

Answer

(a) A congenital defect of platelet function, most likely thrombasthenia.

(b) Platelet aggregation studies.

Discussion

In view of the normal coagulation tests and platelet count and the gross prolongation of the bleeding time, the most likely diagnosis is an inherited defect of platelet function. Since the blood film is stated to be normal it is clear that platelet size and staining characteristics are normal. This, together with the severity of the bleeding defect, makes thrombasthenia the most likely diagnosis. Bernard–Soulier syndrome and the May–Hegglin anomaly are excluded by the normal-sized platelets and the grey platelet syndrome is excluded by the normal size and staining characteristics of the platelets.

The most useful test in establishing a diagnosis would be platelet aggregation studies. In thrombasthenia there may be some aggregation with ristocetin but there is no aggregation with adrenaline, ADP or collagen. The inheritance of thrombasthenia is autosomal recessive, so the lack of a family history is to be expected.

Question 12

Answer

(a) Von Willebrand's disease.

(b) Any two of: platelet aggregation; assay of von Willebrand's antigen; assay of the ristocetin cofactor.

Discussion

The combination of a prolonged bleeding time and a reduced factor VIII concentration is strongly suggestive of von Willebrand's disease. Any of the tests listed would be useful in confirmation. Platelet aggregation is normal with adrenaline, ADP and collagen but is reduced with ristocetin. This abnormality is consequent on a reduction of von Willebrand's factor in the plasma and can be quantified by a ristocetin cofactor assay. In contrast with haemophilia, von Willebrand's antigen (previously referred to as factor-VIII-related antigen) is reduced. Its concentration is similar to the concentration of factor VIII.

Question 13

Answer

(a) Pernicious anaemia.

(b) Schilling test (Parts I and II).

(c) Assay for intrinsic factor antibodies.

(d) Shift of red cell iron into the reticuloendothelial system.

Discussion

A macrocytic anaemia with leucopenia, thrombocytopenia and a significant reduction of the serum vitamin B_{12} concentration in an elderly woman is most suggestive of pernicious anaemia, particularly when there is also numbness of the toes. Some reduction of the red cell folate concentration is common in vitamin B_{12} deficiency.

The diagnosis can be confirmed by a Schilling test which shows vitamin B_{12} malabsorption, correctable with intrinsic factor. "Investigation of vitamin B_{12} absorption" or a "Dicopac test" would also be correct answers, although the proprietary Dicopac test is less satisfactory than a two-part Schilling test in ascertaining the cause of vitamin B_{12} deficiency.

The detection of intrinsic factor antibodies would also confirm the diagnosis, although positive results are not obtained in all patients. Intrinsic factor antibodies are very rare in patients without pernicious anaemia although they have occasionally been detected in patients with autoimmune thyroid disease. In the patient described they would be confirmatory of a diagnosis of pernicious anaemia. Detection of intrinsic factor antibodies will avoid the need to do a Schilling test in some patients. When no antibodies are detected a Schilling test should be performed.

A bone marrow aspirate would be a less satisfactory answer to questions (a) and (b). Although it might well be performed in order to confirm the presence of a megaloblastic anaemia, it would not provide a specific diagnosis.

The serum ferritin is elevated because as the haemoglobin concentration falls there is a shift of haemoglobin from red cells into macrophages.

Question 14

Answer

Self-administration of warfarin.

Discussion

A likely explanation is surreptitious self-administration of warfarin. The patient appears to have an acquired coagulation defect without any evidence of liver disease or disseminated intravascular coagulation. The coagulation defect is suggestive of either vitamin K deficiency or an oral anticoagulant effect. The patient is said to have a good diet and has no symptoms of malabsorption. Surreptitious self-administration of oral anticoagulants usually occurs in those with ready access to these drugs, e.g. nurses, and sometimes in individuals for whom anticoagulants have previously been prescribed.

An alternative explanation would be vitamin K deficiency, for example consequent on coeliac disease. Although there are no features in the history to support this possibility, it should nevertheless be included in the differential diagnosis.

A lupus anticoagulant could be considered as an explanation of a coagulopathy in a patient with a previous history of a pulmonary embolus but the history of nosebleeds and bruising is more suggestive of a coagulopathy than of a lupus anticoagulant which is not associated with a bleeding tendency, and the correction of clotting tests on mixing with fresh normal plasma suggests a clotting factor deficiency rather than an inhibitor of coagulation.

Further Reading

Wallach, J. (1994). "Laboratory diagnosis of factitious disorders", *Arch. Intern. Med.* **154**, 1690–1696.

Question 15

Answer

(a) Lead poisoning.

(b) Serum lead concentration.

Discussion

The anaemia, increased serum bilirubin and increased reticulocyte count suggest a haemolytic anaemia. Haemolytic anaemia with basophilic stippling and a history of constipation is suggestive of lead poisoning. Lead poisoning can also cause a microcytic anaemia. The diagnosis can be confirmed by a serum lead level.

Question 16

Answer

(a) Multiple myeloma.

(b) Bone marrow aspiration (possibly supplemented by trephine biopsy); a test for urinary Bence–Jones protein; skeletal survey including skull X-ray.

(c) Correction of dehydration; correction of hypercalcaemia, e.g. by rehydration, frusemide, corticosteroids and biphosphonates.

Discussion

The bone pain, lytic lesions, hypercalcaemia and hypogammaglobulinaemia suggest a diagnosis of multiple myeloma. The slight elevation of the ESR and the lack of a serum paraprotein make the most likely diagnosis Bence–Jones myeloma. Non-secretory myeloma is also possible but is much less common than Bence–Jones myeloma. It is important to remember that a normal of near-normal ESR does not exclude a diagnosis of multiple myeloma. A normal bone scan is also compatible with multiple myeloma since there is usually no osteoblastic reaction. In contrast to metastatic carcinoma, X-rays are much more sensitive than a bone scan as a means of detecting myelomatous lesions. Similarly, the alkaline phosphatase is usually normal when hypercalcaemia is due to multiple myeloma, the exception being when there is a healing fracture.

The diagnosis should be revealed by a bone marrow aspirate in both Bence–Jones myeloma and non-secretory myeloma while electrophoresis of a concentrated urine specimen is important in the diagnosis of Bence–Jones myeloma. A full skeletal survey is a useful supplementary investigation, the lytic lesions in the skull being the most specific radiological sign of multiple myeloma.

The important therapeutic measures are those directed at correcting the dehydration and hypercalcaemia. This is likely to lead to correction of the renal impairment. Pain relief is also very important. Allopurinol should be administered. Chemotherapy is of secondary importance in the immediate management of the patient.

Question 17

Answer

(a) Pseudo or "stress" polycythaemia.

(b) Cigarette smoking.

Discussion

The red cell mass is within normal limits (although towards the upper limit of normal) whereas the plasma volume is reduced. This is indicative of pseudopolycythaemia. Total red cell mass and plasma volume are best expressed in terms of predictions for a patient's height and weight, but since this patient is not obese a valid interpretation can also be given for results expressed as ml/kg. Polycythaemia rubra vera or primary proliferative polycythaemia would be a wrong answer, and "polycythaemia" would be an inadequate answer.

In many cases the cause of pseudopolycythaemia cannot be determined. Diuretics can be excluded in this patient, since he is said to be taking no drugs. The most likely cause is cigarette smoking, which may also be responsible for the elevated neutrophil count and white cell count. Cigarette smoking can cause not only true polycythaemia, consequent on elevated concentrations of carboxyhaemoglobin or on chronic obstructive lung disease, but also pseudopolycythaemia consequent on reduced plasma volume.

Further Reading

Bain, B. J. (1992). "Haematological effects of smoking", *J. Smoking Rel. Disorders* **3**, 99–108.

Question 18

Answer

(a) The most likely cause of the thrombocytopenia is heparin.

(b) Heparin should be stopped.

(c) Post-transfusion purpura.

Discussion

The coagulation tests are consistent with a heparin effect and show no evidence of disseminated intravascular coagulation. Thrombocytopenia associated with arterial thrombosis with an onset ten days after starting therapy suggests heparin-induced thrombocytopenia.

Heparin causes thrombocytopenia by two mechanisms. Firstly, it can cause mild thrombocytopenia with an onset within three days, which is reversible despite continuing therapy and does not have an immunological basis. Secondly, it can cause more severe thrombocytopenia with an onset between 5 and 15 days associated with arterial and venous thrombosis. The latter type of heparin-induced thrombocytopenia is immune in origin, antibodies probably being directed at a heparin-platelet factor 4 complex and leading to platelet aggregation and venous and arterial thrombosis. Heparin should be stopped immediately. If there is a continuing need for anticoagulation an alternative should be used, e.g. low molecular weight heparin (often there is no cross-reaction), a heparin substitute (such as a mixture of heparan sulphate and dermatan sulphate), warfarin or aspirin.

Thrombocytopenia consequent of platelet alloantibodies should also be considered in the differential diagnosis of thrombocytopenia with an onset ten days after major surgery (which is likely to have been associated with blood transfusion). Such alloantibodies cause destruction also of autologous platelets. However, this syndrome would not provide an explanation of a brachial artery thrombosis in an adequately anticoagulated patient.

Further Reading

Amiral, J.; Wolf, M.; Fischer, A.-M.; Boyer-Neuman, C.; Vissac, A.-M.; Meyer. D. (1996). "Pathogenicity of IgA and/or IgM antibodies to heparin-PF4 complexes in patients with heparin-induced thrombocytopenia", *Brit. J. Haematol.* **92**, 954–959.

Question 19

Answer

Chronic myelomonocytic leukaemia.

Discussion

The most likely diagnosis is chronic myelomonocytic leukaemia, which is classified as one of the myelodysplastic syndromes. Myelodysplastic syndrome, or MDS, would also be a correct answer.

The patient has neutrophilia and monocytosis with a mild thrombocytopenia and a mild macrocytic anaemia which does not appear to be explained by vitamin B_{12} or folate deficiency, liver disease or hypothyroidism. The blood film shows dysplastic features including hypogranular and hypolobulated neutrophils. Macrocytosis is common in the myelodysplastic syndromes.

The blood count does not show the features expected in Philadelphia-positive chronic granulocytic leukaemia since there is no eosinophilia or basophilia and the monocyte count is disproportionately raised in relation to the neutrophil count. Chronic myeloid leukaemia would be a less satisfactory answer than chronic myelomonocytic leukaemia because it is a less specific diagnosis but would not be wrong and would attract some marks.

Question 20

Answer

(a) Parvovirus B19.

(b) Investigation for Parvovirus B19 DNA in serum.

(c) Blood transfusion; high dose intravenous immunoglobulin.

Discussion

The peripheral blood count shows a marked reduction in the haemoglobin concentration without an equivalent reduction in the neutrophil count or platelet count. The reticulocyte count is very low, indicating that this is an aregenerative anaemia (i.e. anaemia due to failure of bone marrow output). The bone marrow findings are those of pure red cell aplasia. In a patient with AIDS this is likely to be due to chronic infection with parvovirus B19.

Only patients with defective immunity are likely to develop chronic parvovirus infection leading to chronic red cell aplasia. Such patients do not usually have detectable antiviral antibodies, and diagnosis therefore depends on detection of viral DNA in serum, for example by dot blot hybridization.

Blood transfusion, although likely to be necessary, is only a short term measure. Administration of high dose intravenous immunoglobulin leads to clearance of the virus and recovery of haemopoiesis. If relapse occurs further courses can be given. It should be noted, however, that some patients develop a rash, arthritis and an elevated ESR after administration of immunoglobulin.

Further Reading

French, A. L.; Sacks, L.; Schechter, G. P. (1996). "Fifth disease after immunoglobulin administration in an AIDS patient with Parvovirus-induced red cell aplasia", *Am. J. Med.* **101**, 108–109.

PHOTOGRAPHS

(1) Bone marrow aspirate.

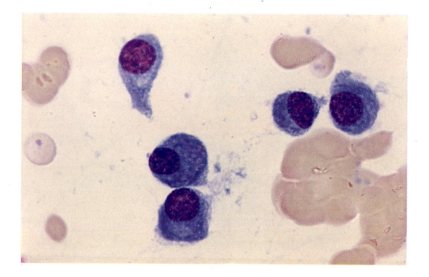

What is the diagnosis?

....

(2) Iron stain of a bone marrow aspirate.

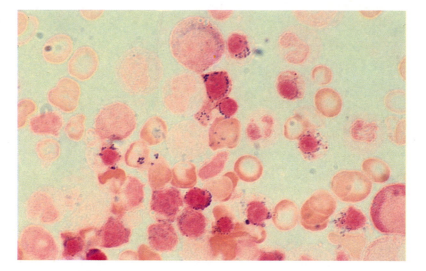

(a) What is the most significant abnormality?

....

(b) List two possible causes.

....

....

(3) Blood film of a 44-year-old West Indian patient with generalized lymphadenopathy, lymphocytosis, a negative Paul–Bunnell test and hypercalcaemia.

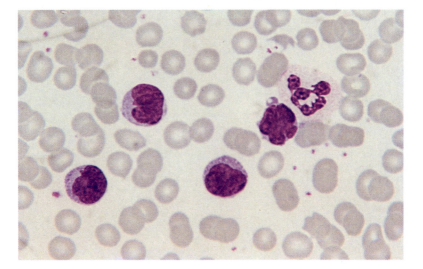

(a) What is the most likely diagnosis?

....

(b) What two tests would you do to confirm the diagnosis?

....

....

(4) Blood film.

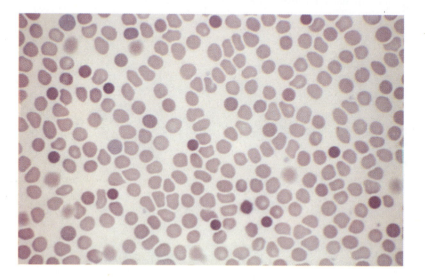

(a) What is the most significant abnormality?

....

(b) List two causes of this abnormality.

....

....

(5) Blood film of a six-year-old Cypriot boy who presented with the sudden onset of symptoms of anaemia. He was receiving treatment for a urinary tract infection.

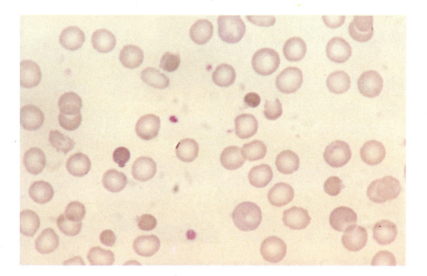

What is the likely diagnosis?

....

(6) Bone marrow aspirate of a 60-year-old male smoker with a cough and weight loss.

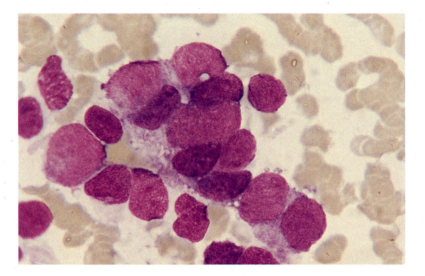

What is the most likely diagnosis?

....

(7) Blood film.

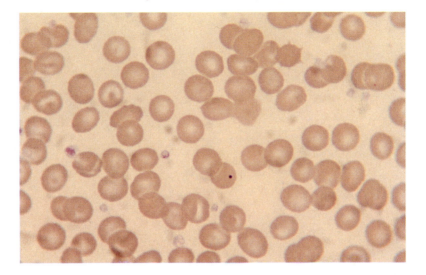

(a) List the three most significant abnormalities.

....

....

....

(b) What does this combination of abnormalities indicate?

....

(8) Blood film of a patient with a lifelong bleeding disorder.

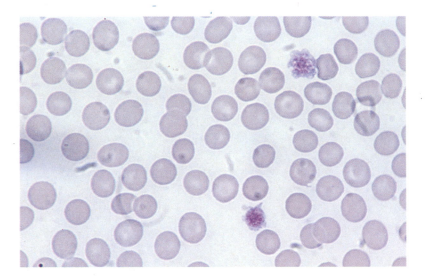

(a) What is the most significant abnormality?

....

(b) What is the most likely diagnosis?

....

(9) Blood film.

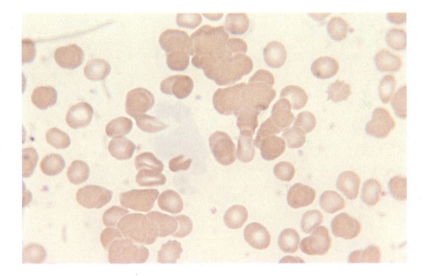

(a) What is the most significant abnormality?

....

(b) List two illnesses which could cause this abnormality.

....

....

(10) Blood film of a 65-year-old woman with weight loss, indigestion and anaemia.

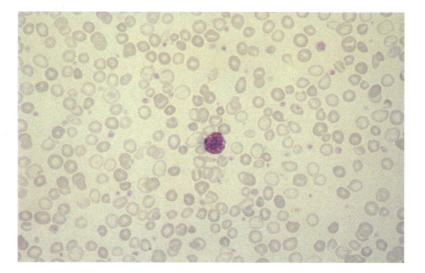

(a) List the two most significant abnormalities.

....

....

(b) What is the most likely cause of the anaemia?

....

(11) Bone marrow aspirate of a five-year-old child with pallor and bruising.

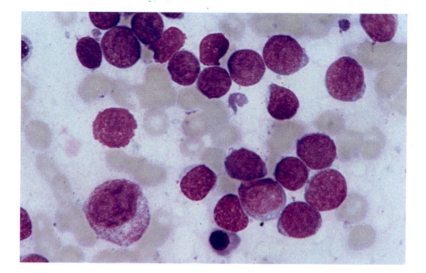

What is the likely diagnosis?

....

(12) Blood film of a 40-year-old man with marked splenomegaly.

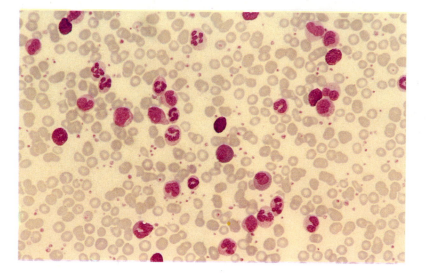

(a)   What is the most likely diagnosis?

    ....

(b)   What single test would be most useful in confirming the diagnosis?

    ....

(13) Skull X-ray.

(a) What is the diagnosis?

....

(b) What is the radio-opacity at the centre of the skull at the level of orbits?

....

(14) Bone marrow from an African child with a jaw tumour and cervical lymphadenopathy.

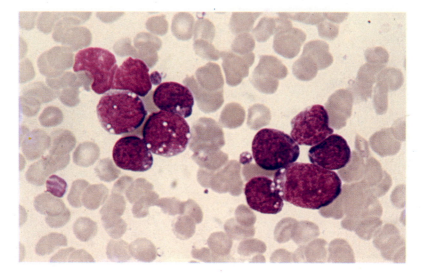

(a)   What is the diagnosis?

      ....

(b)   What virus has been implicated in the aetiology of this condition?

      ....

(15) Photograph of an arm.

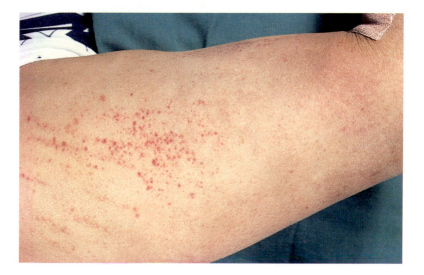

(a) What abnormality is shown?

....

(b) List two possible causes.

....

....

(16) Blood film of a Ghanaian patient.

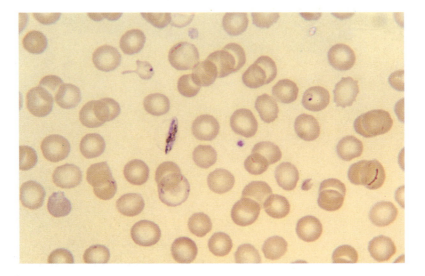

What is the diagnosis?

....

(17) Blood film of a Nigerian patient.

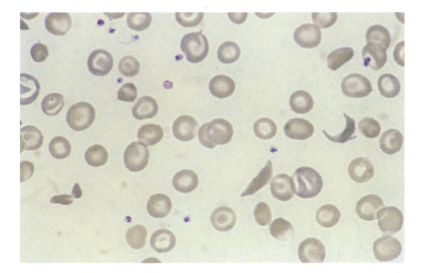

What is the most likely diagnosis?

....

(18) Blood film of a febrile North African child.

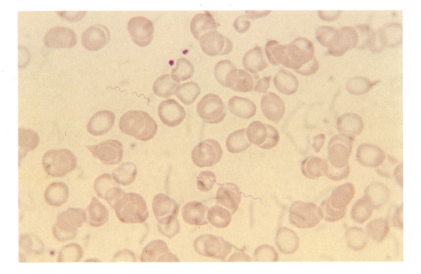

(a) What micro-organisms are present?

....

(b) What illness would the child be suffering from?

....

(19) Blood film of a 50-year-old woman with pallor, bruising and slight splenomegaly.

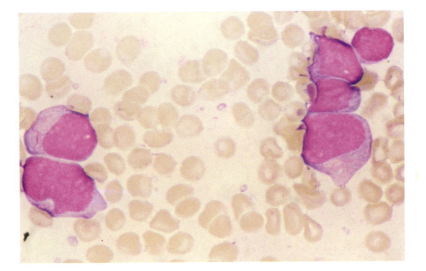

What is the most likely diagnosis?

....

(20) Blood film.

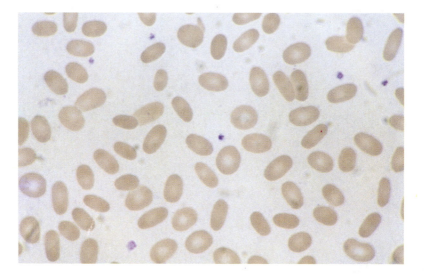

(a) What is the diagnosis?

....

(b) Is this condition usually of any clinical significance?

....

(21) Blood film of a febrile West African.

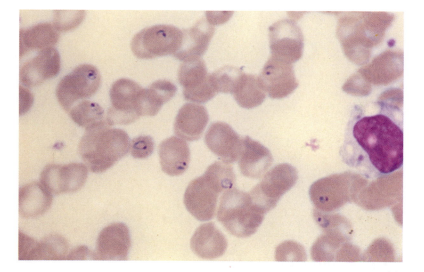

What is the diagnosis?

....

(22, 23) Blood film and clinical photo of a 68-year-old Caucasian male.

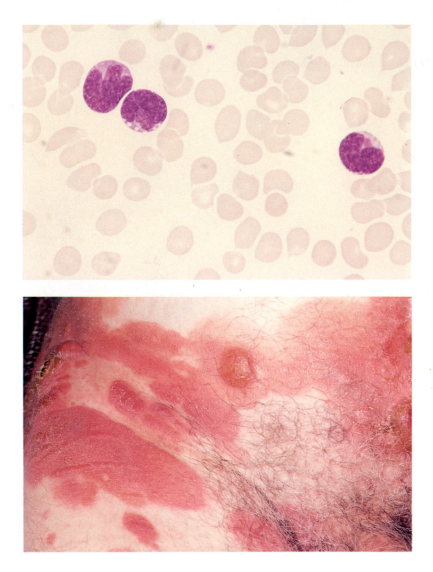

What is the most likely diagnosis?

....

(24) Blood film of a 23-year-old male engineering student with fever, malaise, cervical lymphadenopathy and mild jaundice.

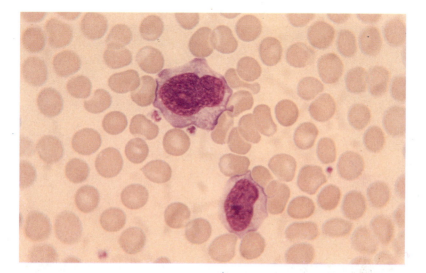

What is the most likely diagnosis?

....

(25) Abdominal CT scan of a 45-year-old male with abdominal discomfort and weight loss. The scan was performed after the administration of intravenous and oral contrast media.

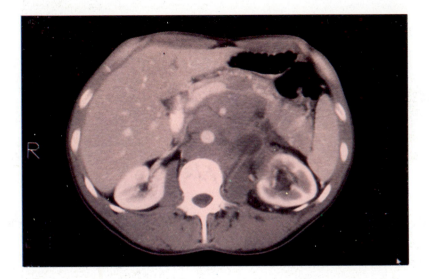

(a)   What is the most likely diagnosis?

....

(b)   What abnormality is shown by the left kidney?

....

(26, 27) Hand and foot of a 70-year-old woman with rheumatoid arthritis.

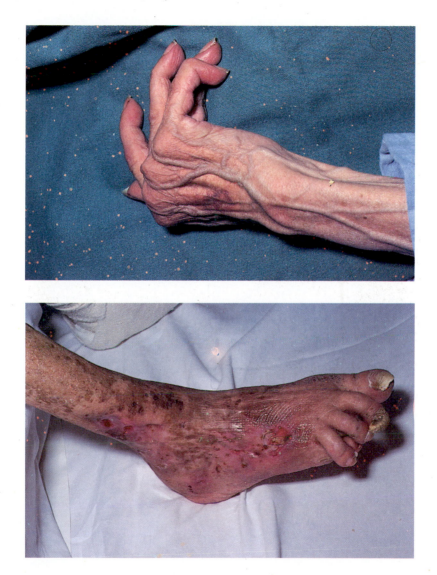

What is the most likely diagnosis?

....

(28) Blood film of a Sri Lankan patient.

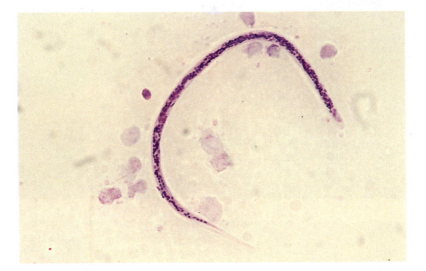

What is the diagnosis?

....

(29) Bone marrow aspirate film of a Spanish man with AIDS.

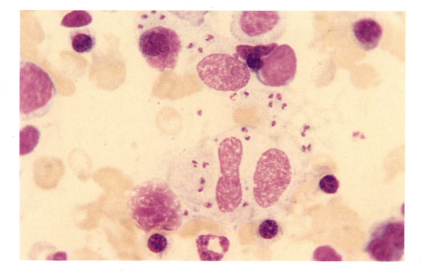

What is the diagnosis?

....

(30) Bone marrow aspirate of a patient with splenomegaly and a very slowly progressive pancytopenia.

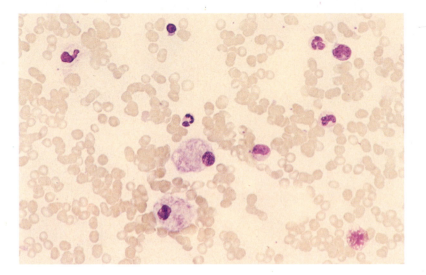

What is the diagnosis?

....

(31) Bone marrow aspirate of a two-year-old child with emaciation, psychomotor retardation, spasticity and blindness.

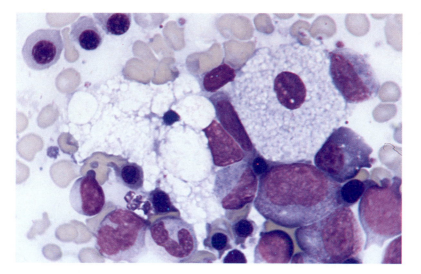

(a)   What abnormality is shown?

....

(b)   What is the most likely diagnosis?

....

(32) Blood film of a patient with dermatitis herpetiformis.

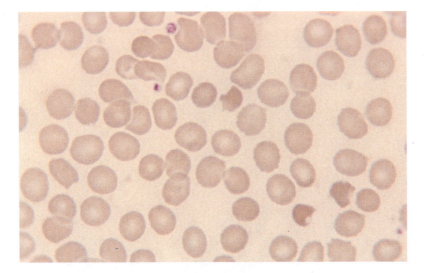

What drug is the patient likely to be taking?

....

(33) Leg of a patient who is neutropenic following chemotherapy.

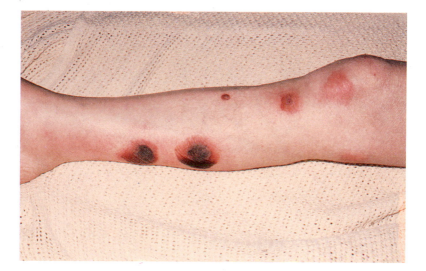

What is the likely diagnosis?

....

(34) Blood film of a healthy Italian woman with a normal haemoglobin concentration.

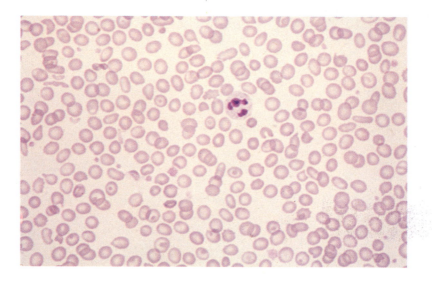

(a)   List the four most significant abnormalities shown.

....

....

....

....

(b)   What is the most likely diagnosis?

....

(35) Photograph of hands.

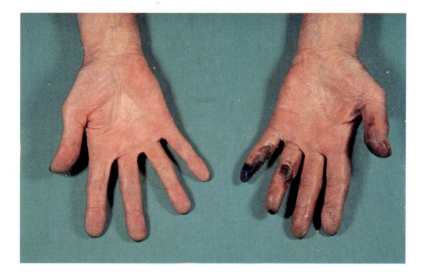

List three haematological disorders which could cause this abnormality.

....

....

....

(36) Photograph of a patient's mouth.

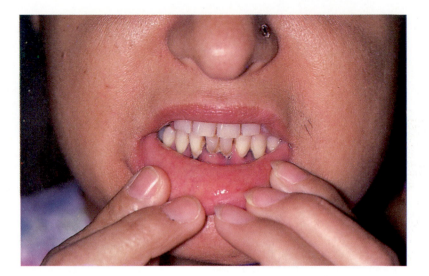

What is the diagnosis?

....

(37) Blood film of an anaemic patient.

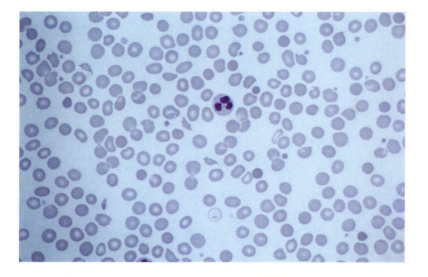

(a) List two significant abnormalities.

....

....

(b) What is this type of anaemia called?

....

(38) Blood film of a West African patient.

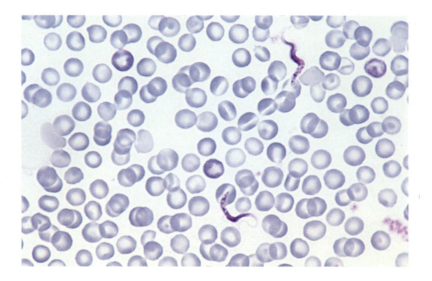

What is the diagnosis?

....

(39) Trephine biopsy from a patient with severe pancytopenia.

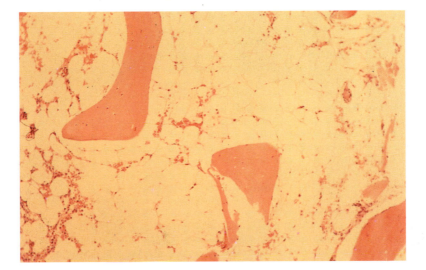

What is the diagnosis?

....

(40) CT scan of a patient with a leucoerythroblastic blood film and intermittent claudication.

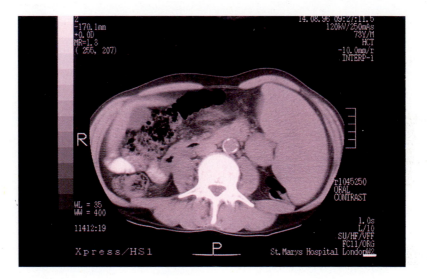

List two likely diagnoses (one being responsible for the leucoerythroblastic anaemia and the other being incidental).

....

....

PHOTOGRAPHS
ANSWERS AND DISCUSSION

Question 1

Answer

Multiple myeloma.

Discussion

The normal bone marrow cells have been replaced by plasma cells which are recognized by their eccentric nuclei, marked cytoplasmic basophilia and the Golgi zones which are apparent in some cells.

Question 2

Answer

(a) Numerous ring sideroblasts.

(b) Congenital sideroblastic anaemia; primary acquired sideroblastic anaemia.

Discussion

This patient had primary acquired sideroblastic anaemia, also known as refractory anaemia with ring sideroblasts, which is one of the myelodysplastic syndromes. Congenital sideroblastic anaemia is also associated with large numbers of sideroblasts. Other causes of ring sideroblasts, usually in smaller numbers, include exposure to alcohol and to certain drugs, such as anti-tuberculous drugs.

Question 3

Answer

(a) Adult T-cell leukaemia/lymphoma.

(b) Serology for HTLV-I (the human T-cell leukaemia virus); immunophenotyping of abnormal cells to demonstrate that they are T-cells.

Discussion

The blood film shows very abnormal lymphoid cells with lobulated nuclei. The lymphocyte adjacent to the neutrophil has a flower-shaped nucleus. The fact that the patient in West Indian and has lymphadenopathy and hypercalcaemia suggests this diagnosis. The causative virus, HTLV-I, is also endemic in the south-eastern United States and in Japan. (Note: although this particular question may be a little too difficult for MRCP, it is important for physicians to be familiar with this virus and with the spectrum of diseases with which it is associated.)

Question 4

Answer

(a) Spherocytosis.

(b) Hereditary spherocytosis; autoimmune haemolytic anaemia.

Discussion

These are the only two common causes of spherocytosis. Rare causes include haemolytic disease of the newborn, delayed transfusion reactions and *Clostridium welchii* septicaemia.

Question 5

Answer

Glucose-6-phosphate dehydrogenase (G6PD) deficiency.

Discussion

The film confirms that the patient is anaemic and shows a number of irregularly contracted cells. These are consequent on oxidation of haemoglobin. In G6PD deficiency the red cells are not protected against oxidant stress, for example due to infection or exposure to certain drugs, and denaturation of haemoglobin and haemolysis occurs. G6PD deficiency is common among Cypriot males.

Question 6

Answer

Metastatic small cell carcinoma of the lung (oat cell carcinoma).

Discussion

The bone marrow aspirate shows a clump of non-haemopoietic malignant cells. The history suggests that this is likely to be metastatic lung cancer. The cytological features are also typical, there being moulding of nuclei by the nuclei of adjacent cells.

Question 7

Answer

(a) Target cells, a Howell–Jolly body and an acanthocyte.

(b) Hyposplenism.

Discussion

Only hyposplenism causes this particular combination of abnormalities. Other peripheral blood features of hyposplenism may include lymphocytosis, thrombocytosis, large platelets and occasional spherocytes.

Question 8

Answer

(a) Giant platelets.

(b) Bernard–Soulier syndrome or another of the congenital thrombocytopenias with giant platelets.

Discussion

The blood film shows thrombocytopenia and giant platelets. The May–Hegglin anomaly also has this combination of features, but neither the thrombocytopenia nor the macrothrombocytosis is as marked as in Bernard–Soulier syndrome and neutrophils show characteristic inclusions.

Question 9

Answer

(a) Red cell agglutinates.

(b) Pneumonia caused by *Mycoplasma pneumoniae*; chronic cold haemagglutinin disease.

Discussion

Red cell agglutinates in a blood film indicate the presence of a cold agglutinin. This is quite common in patients without any apparent relevant illness. However, the question asks which illnesses could cause this abnormality. Recognized causes include acute infections, such as those due to *Mycoplasma pneumoniae* or the Epstein–Barr virus (infectious mononucleosis), or chronic lymphoproliferative disorders such as chronic cold haemagglutinin disease.

Question 10

Answer

(a) Hypochromia and microcytosis.

(b) Iron deficiency.

Discussion

The film also shows anisocytosis, anisochromasia and mild poikilocytosis but it is the hypochromia and microcytosis which are the most significant features because they suggest a relevant differential diagnosis. In view of the patient's history iron deficiency anaemia is most likely.

Question 11

Answer

Acute lymphoblastic leukaemia.

Discussion

The film shows one nucleated red cell and one granulocyte precursor but all the other cells are blast cells. In view of the age of the child this is most likely acute lymphoblastic leukaemia and, in fact, the cytological features of the blast cells are typical of lymphoblasts.

Question 12

Answer

(a) Chronic granulocytic leukaemia.

(b) Cytogenetic analysis to detect the Philadelphia chromosome.

Discussion

The blood film shows leukocytosis with myeloid cells at all stages of maturation. This plus the history of marked splenomegaly suggests that this is chronic rather than acute myeloid leukaemia. Cytogenetic analysis to detect the specific translocation, t(9;22), which is associated with this type of leukaemia is the best test to do, because it is most specific. Tests such as the neutrophil alkaline phosphatase (which is characteristically lowered) are less specific.

Question 13

Answer

(a) Multiple myeloma.

(b) A hearing aid.

Discussion

The skull radiograph shows multiple punched-out lytic lesions typical of multiple myeloma. It is important to recognize extraneous objects such as hearing aids in X-rays so that they are not confused with pathological lesions.

Question 14

Answer

(a) Burkitt's lymphoma.

(b) The Epstein–Barr virus.

Discussion

The diagnosis can be strongly suspected from the history and is confirmed by the presence of blast cells with very basophilic cytoplasm and vacuolated cytoplasma, the hallmarks of Burkitt's lymphoma.

Question 15

Answer

(a) Petechiae.

(b) Severe thrombocytopenia or self-induced injury.

Discussion

The photograph shows petechiae (pin-point cutaneous haemorrhages), some of which are in straight lines. Linear haemorrhagic lesions suggest the possibility of deliberate self-induced injury. However, this patient had severe thrombocytopenia and the petechiae are linear because she happened to scratch her arm when her platelet count was very low.

Question 16

Answer

Plasmodium falciparum malaria.

Discussion

The film shows a crescent-shaped gametocyte, so *Plasmodium falciparum* malaria is the only possible diagnosis.

Question 17

Answer

Sickle cell anaemia.

Discussion

The film shows that the patient is anaemic. Sickle cells and target cells are present. The most likely diagnosis is sickle cell anaemia (homozygosity for haemoglobin S).

Question 18

Answer

(a) Borrelia.

(b) Borreliosis or relapsing fever.

Discussion

The spiral organisms present are *Borrelia* species, which, unlike most spiral organisms, are visible on routinely stained blood films.

Question 19

Answer

Acute myeloid leukaemia.

Discussion

The blood film shows numerous blast cells. The presence of fine cytoplasmic granules suggests that these are myeloblasts, and this is confirmed by the presence of an Auer rod, a crystalline cytoplasmic inclusion, in one of the blast cells. Leucocytosis with a predominance of blast cells is indicative of acute rather than chronic myeloid leukaemia.

Question 20

Answer

(a) Hereditary elliptocytosis.

(b) No.

Discussion

A blood film with such a large number of elliptocytes and ovalocytes is diagnostic of hereditary elliptocytosis. It is uncommon for hereditary elliptocytosis to be associated with anaemia or even with significant haemolysis.

Question 21

Answer

Plasmodium falciparum malaria.

Discussion

The film shows numerous very fine ring forms of *Plasmodium falciparum*. The only other malaria which is common in West Africa is *Plasmodium ovale*, which has much larger ring forms in enlarged and decolourized red cells.

Questions 22 and 23

Answer

Mycosis fungoides.

Discussion

Either mycosis fungoides or Sézary syndrome would be a correct diagnosis. The blood film shows large atypical lymphocytes with very irregular nuclei (Séary cells). The photograph of the inguinal region shows plaque-like infiltration and fungating lesions. Mycosis fungoides is the only disease which is likely to cause this combination of abnormalities. Immunophenotyping showed that, as expected, the atypical cells were T-cells.

Question 24

Answer

Infectious mononucleosis.

Discussion

The blood film shows atypical lymphocytes (also referred to as atypical mononuclear cells). These are larger than normal lymphocytes with irregular nuclei and plentiful cytoplasm which shows peripheral basophilia. There is "scalloping" of lymphocytes around adjacent red cells. These features and the patient's history are typical of infectious mononucleosis. Glandular fever would also be a correct answer.

Question 25

Answer

(a) Non-Hodgkin's lymphoma.

(b) Hydronephrosis.

Discussion

The CT scan shows a large mass of para-aortic and mesenteric lymph nodes, displacing the aorta and the bowel. The left kidney is hydronephrotic, suggesting that the ureter is obstructed by lymph nodes. The combination of the history and the CT scan suggests non-Hodgkin's lymphoma. Biopsy showed follicular lymphoma. Hodgkin's disease could be an explanation for para-aortic lymphadenopathy but would not be expected to cause bulky mesenteric lymphadenopathy.

Questions 26 and 27

Answer

Hyperviscosity syndrome.

Discussion

The hand shows ulnar deviation of rheumatoid arthritis and gross venous distension. The foot shows severe circulatory impairment. The venous distension and impaired circulation were consequent on a hyperviscousity syndrome caused by very high levels of rheumatoid factor. This is an uncommon complication of rheumatoid arthritis.

Question 28

Answer

Filariasis.

Discussion

The parasite shown in *Wucheria bancrofti*. It is distinguishable from other microfilaria, in that the nuclei do not extend into the tip of the tail. The body nuclei are coarse and well separated and the head space is as long as it is broad.

Question 29

Answer

Leishmaniasis.

Discussion

The bone marrow shows numerous Leishman–Donovan bodies which are identified by the double dot of the nucleus and the kinetoplast in each organism. Leishmaniasis occurs around the Mediterranean and has an increased incidence in patients with AIDS.

Question 30

Answer

Gaucher's disease.

Discussion

The bone marrow aspirate shows two Gaucher's cells. They are very large cells with cytoplasm which has been described as resembling watered silk.

Question 31

Answer

(a) Two foamy macrophages.

(b) Niemann–Pick disease.

Discussion

The bone marrow shows two foam cells, i.e. macrophages distended with lipid vacuoles. There are a number of causes of foamy macrophages in the bone marrow but, given the clinical features, Nieman–Pick disease is the most likely in this child.

Question 32

Answer

Dapsone.

Discussion

The film shows irregularly contracted cells. These are characteristic of oxidant damage to red cells. Dapsone, which is commonly used in the treatment of dermatitis herpetiformis, is an oxidant drug which often causes red cell damage, even in people without G6PD deficiency. Haemoglobin is denatured to methaemoglobin with formation of Heinz bodies which are pitted from red cells by the spleen. If haemolysis is very acute a Heinz body preparation is positive.

Question 33

Answer

Pseudomonas infection.

Discussion

These black lesions are so chacteristic of Pseudomonas infection that the diagnosis can be suspected on clinical examination before results of cultures are obtained.

Question 34

Answer

(a) Hypochromia; microcytosis; poikilocytosis; target cells.

(b) Beta thalassaemia trait.

Discussion

The film also shows anisocytosis but this is a very non-specific feature. The poikilocytes present include tear-drop poikilocytes and elliptocytes but target cells are more numerous and more important in diagnosis. Microcytosis and poikilocytosis with the presence of target cells in a healthy young Italian with a normal haemoglobin suggest beta thalassaemia trait. Hypochromia is not always present in beta thalassaemia trait but it is apparent in this patient.

Question 35

Answer

Polycythaemia rubra vera (primary proliferative polycythaemia); essential thrombocythaemia; cryoglobulinaemia.

Discussion

The fingers, particularly the tips, are ischaemic. This could be consequent on vascular obstruction caused by hyperviscosity from polycythaemia rubra vera, a high platelet count in essential thrombocythaemia or precipitation of cryoglobulinaemia in cryoglobulinaemia. In this particular patient the cause was polycythaemia rubra vera. Other correct answers would include other causes of hyperviscosity, e.g. Waldenström's macroglobulinaemia.

Question 36

Answer

Lead poisoning.

Discussion

The photograph shows a lead line and is diagnostic of lead poisoning.

Question 37

Answer

(a) Spherocytes or microspherocytes; red cell fragments (or schistocytes).

(b) Microangiopathic haemolytic anaemia.

Question 38

Answer

Trypanosomiasis.

Discussion

The parasite shown is actually *Trypanosoma brucei gambesiense* but this cannot be distinguished from *Trypanosoma brucei rhodesiense* on morphology alone.

Question 39

Answer

Aplastic anaemia.

Discussion

The trephine biopsy shows that bone marrow haemopoietic cells have been largely replaced by fat. It should be noted that despite the designation "aplastic anaemia" this condition leads to pancytopenia rather than just anaemia.

Question 40

Answer

Idiopathic myelofibrosis; atherosclerosis.

Discussion

The scan shows gross splenic enlargement. This, together with a leucoerythroblastic blood film, suggests that the patient has idiopathic myelofibrosis, also referred to as myelofibrosis with myeloid metaplasia.

The scan also shows calcification of the aorta. This plus the history of intermittent claudication suggests that the patient has atherosclerosis.